PLAYING

DOCTOR

FROM THE BOARDS
TO THE WARDS

PLAYING DOCTOR
FROM THE BOARDS TO THE WARDS

Copyright © 2016
Written by Emilee Sandsmark
Edited by Evan Sandsmark

Cover photo Alex Benison
Cover design Eric Nelson

Table of Contents

ACKNOWLEDGEMENTS..I

DEDICATION III

PREVIEW..V

PROLOGUE i

CHAPTER 1 1

CHAPTER 2...4

CHAPTER 3...10

CHAPTER 4...16

CHAPTER 5...27

CHAPTER 6...35

CHAPTER 7...52

CHAPTER 8...61

CHAPTER 9...80

CHAPTER 10...91

CHAPTER 11...102

CHAPTER 12...113

CHAPTER 13...125

CHAPTER 14...145

CHAPTER 15...157

CHAPTER 16...165

CHAPTER 17...176

CHAPTER 18...186

CHAPTER 19...190

CHAPTER 20...196

CHAPTER 21...207

CHAPTER 22...212

ACKNOWLEDGEMENTS

I have many people to acknowledge in the making of this book. The biggest thank you of all goes to my brother, **Evan Sandsmark**, who was the primary editor. With his dedication, intelligence, and talent, I am able to give off the illusion that I am capable of writing a book. He made this possible for me.

There are several other people that contributed significantly, and without their input and advice, this book would not be the same. I greatly appreciate all the hard work of **Gabe Wilner, Lorna Bremner, and Joanna Sandsmark**.

I also want to thank **Alex Benison** for the cover photo and **Eric Nelson** for the cover design.

DEDICATION

My memoir is dedicated to my dearest fellow CU school of medicine friends: **Josi Schwan, Lauren Harrington, Racheal Gilmer, Lauren Nading, Monica Davern, and Feven Tesfeladit**—a.k.a. Brad, Bruce, Howard, Dennis, Kevin and Sebastian, respectively. (Inside joke. Don't worry about it.) I would not be where I am today without your invaluable, unconditional support. While the words "thank you" will never be enough to do my gratitude justice, I hope a dedication in a book helps. (And really, what more could you ask for?)
Love, Spike

The nature of this book naturally draws me to dedicate it to my medical school friends, but equally as essential and appreciated are my friends outside of school and my family. Let's face it, I wasn't always the best of friends or family members to all of you and you all continued to be there for me to see me through my journey. You know who you are, and now with this, I hope you are reminded that I love and appreciate you more than I can express with words.

PREVIEW

I stood in the OR with lead in my shoes. This was only the second crash C-section I had ever observed. I was scared for everyone in the room, including myself. I desperately wanted to be helpful, but knew this was no place for a medical student. One of the residents looked at me and asked, "Hey Emilee, can you please wait in the hallway with Mr. S?"

I quickly nodded. I had already learned that I should treat all questions as commands. I tried to fake a smile at him and we exited the OR into the hall. My first reaction was, "Wow, now this is an important job to ask of a medical student!" Then my second thought was, "Holy shit!!! Now THIS is an important job to ask of a medical student!!"

What was I supposed to say or do with him? I took one look at the color of his face and quickly searched for a chair, explaining my actions as I went, all the while trying to prepare myself for what seemed an inevitable faint. He assured me he didn't want to sit and started to pace. I could not think of anything obvious to say or do next. Small talk did not seem appropriate, nor did reassurance.

Essentially all I knew at this point was how important this pregnancy was to him and that it could potentially end disastrously, and I would likely be with the father when he first found out. I felt helpless and overwhelmed. I didn't know who would faint first—him or me. Between the two of us, it was a race to the floor.

PROLOGUE

I am the best and I am the worst; I am everything and I am nothing. I am the most laid back, high-strung person you will ever meet. I am inquisitive and ambitious, and yet there are days that I would rather stay in my pajamas on the couch and watch TV or perhaps just stare at the ceiling. I can be very irritable and impatient but have a huge heart filled with compassion and love for people. I am very considerate, and yet altogether selfish. I consider myself non-judgmental, but constantly reprimand myself for being overly critical. I am intelligent, but am frequently in tears because I wanted to do just a little bit better on an exam, leading me to believe I may not be that smart after all. I am habitually filled with self-doubt, yet brimming with confidence. I have never been happier than I have been while in medical school, and yet it is a constant source of turmoil, conflict, and anxiety.

I have been described as all of these things before, and while they are all essentially contradictory, they are all accurate. They vary in their degree of expression and it is the harmony of these attributes that makes me an individual. Fortunately for me, the University of Colorado School of Medicine (CU) recognized that the attributes that (in theory) make a good physician slightly outweighed those that would be a disservice to the profession. I, with all my strengths and weaknesses, was chosen to pursue my calling.

While I was applying to medical school, I thought I was non-traditional. My idea of a traditional applicant was a person who applied to medical school right after college, took the MCAT one time and nailed it, chose difficult coursework and achieved perfect grades, and in general had a resume to rival a future president's. In contrast, I had taken a couple years off from college to bartend and travel. I had to take the MCAT several times before I was satisfied with my score; my grades were good, but by no means perfect; and my resume had a few gaps in it.

I thought my personal background was unique as well. I grew up in rural Colorado with my single mother who always struggled to make ends meet. I felt pride in the fact that I had overcome some adversity, earned good grades, and took the MCAT tirelessly until I had a great score. I thought these attributes made me exceptional, and when I was accepted to medical school, I felt truly special…until I met my classmates. Suddenly my "non-traditional" applicant status seemed anything but in comparison to my fellow classmates.

Upon meeting them, I was constantly in awe of every one of them and frequently felt intimidated to be in their midst. Prior to matriculation, I had become used to admissions essays and interviews, and had perfected a method by which I could elaborate on all of my positive characteristics, spinning all of my drawbacks into assets that contributed to my integrity and tenacity. My MCAT scores, research experience, and educational background were acceptable conversation starters. Yet now, upon meeting my classmates, my MCAT score wasn't the answer to their questions—primarily because it would be absurd for someone to ask for your MCAT score right after meeting you, but also because we all had great MCAT scores. Everyone also had impressive research experience and excellent grades. I was average at best. I had a constant fear that I was far less intelligent and qualified than everyone else. I wasn't accepted to medical school the first year that I tried, so I often wondered whether or not there had been a terrible mistake in letting me into medical school the second time that I had applied.

And apart from the obvious brilliance of my peers, they were *interesting*. My class consisted of a former ship builder, a successful video game programmer, a CIA agent, a lawyer, a couple of PhDs, a professional juggler, and lots of college athletes, to name a few. Here I was thinking I was a "non-traditional" applicant because my parents were divorced, I had grown up in a small town, I was the first doctor in my family, and I took time off between undergraduate and medical school.

Over time, I eventually learned to trust the admissions process and appreciate once again my own background and the distinct assets that I contributed to the class. Eventually, I noticed that I didn't struggle any more than my peers. All of us are completely, but equally, overwhelmed by the colossal amount of material we are asked to learn, and at the end of the day, we all did about the same on our exams. However, I still struggled to appreciate my value when surrounded by amazing people. It is hard to accept being average, and it is equally hard to realize that in medical school excellence is not praised but expected.

I have always been inquisitive. As a child, I made a hobby of asking my parents exhausting and trivial questions, which they often accused me of already knowing the answer to. (I denied it at the time, but looking back it's pretty obvious that I was frequently looking to "confirm" what I already knew.) My parents called such inquiries "busy questions" and I was allowed a certain quota for a particular time period. For instance, during the course of a car ride, I was granted a certain number of "busy questions," and then my mom would say, "Alright, one more busy question for the day and then we are done, okay?" *Ooh, better make this one good,* I would think.

"Do you think Grammy likes ketchup or mustard better?" (I can't imagine why my parents didn't appreciate these provocative questions.) Even more annoyingly, I would often just deliver the standard "why?" after my parents answered me, just as so many other children do. I quickly realized (and found it extremely amusing) that this particular question was appropriate after almost any statement.

I never really grew out of this phase. I am always the one who wants to know who said what, how they said it, who stood where, and why someone chose a turkey sandwich over a ham sandwich for lunch. While I may have exhausted a few family members and friends—okay, I'm *certain* I exhausted them—my relentless questioning serves me well in school.

***

Third year for a medical student is unique, and it is hard to adequately describe to those who don't experience it firsthand, so I will rely on an analogy. Picture yourself lost in a foreign country for a year, and every day you are lost in a different way. Day after day, you have a general destination in mind, but don't know the way to get there. Applying this to the hospital setting, I recognized that our ultimate goal was to diagnose, cure, treat, and alleviate suffering in our patients. However, the means by which we were to achieve these general goals, and what counts as success, were often much less clear.

For instance, in a patient admitted for a cholecystectomy (gallbladder removal), did they need to be pain free before discharge? Was it necessary for them to be able to tolerate solid food, or is okay to let them go home on a liquid diet? I had a very general idea of what we were trying to accomplish, but discerning the details was challenging, just as finding a way to your destination is hard when lost in an unfamiliar city. Initially, you feel overwhelmed, scared, and incompetent. However, as an adult, you have acquired enough skills over your life to take it one step at a time. You know how to read a map, and when the map indicates that you must "take a right on Broadway" or "go north on York," you can start to piece together the directions until you are at your final destination (although inevitably there will be some wrong turns until you finally arrive). Then the next day, you start all over again—a new city, a new destination. Self-doubt bears down on you once more. But again you start managing it bit by bit, and before you know it, you have survived another day.

During the first two years, we are given some of the knowledge and skills to succeed in third year. We learn endless medical facts and are taught how to sift through medical literature for answers, how to perform physical exams, and how to communicate effectively with patients and families. Then third year comes around, the start of our clinical rotations in which we experience many subspecialties and work with an ever-changing group of medical professionals. We are expected to take the medical details that we memorized from books and exams and broadly apply them to the treatment of patients. The emphasis shifts from a microscopic focus to more of a macroscopic one. For a third year student, the big picture is still hard to understand, but we take it one step at a time. Instead of trying to tackle the entire idea of a diabetic hemophiliac with end stage liver disease presenting with acute chest pain, we have to break the problem into smaller pieces using the facts and tools that we were largely taught during the first two years. This is all fine and well, and I can't imagine a more reasonable approach, but the problem for us is that just when we have wrapped ourselves around one patient's history, diagnosis and management, we start all over the next day with an equally daunting and intimidating puzzle, all the while trying to keep a smile on our faces (because our grades depend on it). Even when you've found your destination for the night, a new path awaits tomorrow.

The third year of medical school can be dismaying, but it certainly isn't boring, and that is precisely why I have focused on this year of school and largely this year alone. You might think this is unduly limited, and that some discussion of my first two years would be informative and of some interest. I suppose it could be informative, but I very much doubt it would be of interest. Consider an average day in my life:

I woke up at 6:30AM every day for 8:00AM class. (I forced myself up an hour earlier when my jeans wouldn't button. A workout was no longer an option, but a mandate.) I arrived to class every morning at about 8:07, always sneaking in the back entrance to the large lecture hall. Every day I was just as perplexed as the day prior by my unexpected tardiness. My late arrival didn't really matter, however, because I got right down to business when I settled into my seat. I would pull out my yogurt, my Ziploc bag of granola, and my adorable Tupperware of mixed berries, and then concoct my breakfast, which both entertained and nourished me during the first 15 minutes of class. After that, I would check both my email accounts, then move over to Facebook, and then return to my email accounts. (You never know what could have come in while I was away on Facebook.) I would generally navigate my way to Facebook again for the same reason that I re-checked my email. After this ritual, my Internet browsing varied. I might check my quickly evaporating bank account balance to see if I was truly destitute or merely poor, and I would often check the weather, for no other reason than to know what I would be missing out on while I was studying. By that time, it was hopefully 8:45, meaning the first lecture would be over in 5 minutes.

Playing Doctor

Then it was time for a bathroom break and, if I was feeling bold, a coffee refill. After re-entering the lecture hall at 9:00, I would have a stern conversation with myself about the necessity of paying attention for the next three hours. (Lectures were always from 8:00-12:00.) This self-imposed redirection lasted maybe the next hour (depending on the quality of the lecture), and then the cycle would start all over again, but this time pretzels or nuts accompanied my directionless browsing. Luckily, lectures were recorded, and faculty handouts and notes were graciously provided that adequately compensated for the gaps in my attention. After lectures ended at noon, students basically went their separate ways to study for the afternoon. This is when things got really exciting.

Depending on how I felt, I would either go to the library or return to my apartment to study. (A coffee shop might figure into my study routine as well, but this generally came later in the day.) During the long afternoons and evenings that followed lectures, I basically just studied. Of course, the intensity of my focus waxed and waned, but I was studying just the same, and that is essentially all there is to say. For detail, I suppose I could mention that on occasion I found a diagram particularly helpful or interesting. One day back in November, in the midst of a 14-hour day of preparation for my upcoming metabolism exam, I distinctly recall noting that the print was really clear on the Krebs cycle diagram. I also appreciated the way in which the molecules were depicted, and the legend's placement in the upper-right of the page was well situated for frequent reference. It was an exceptional diagram.

I remember numerous moments like this, when I cursed or praised my books depending on the efficiency with which they crammed information into my brain, and I can imagine few things as boring as my personal reflections on my study materials. The same is true of the debates I had in my head about the optimal time to take a break for eating. (Those blissful 15 minutes chewing my sandwich would only come once – I had to make them count.) The life of the mind is indeed stimulating, but not for those looking from the outside in. So, I'll stick with third year, when the action begins.

While many third year medical students will undoubtedly share similar experiences, I want to stress that this is my story, and only my interpretation of what it takes to become a doctor. I do not wish to generalize my peers' experiences, even though some of our stories are so similar that I was constantly tempted to weave their experiences into my own narrative. I cannot imagine enduring medical school alone, and nothing has been more therapeutic than the times I have spent with fellow students who are also close friends. We often gathered for hours, laughing as we recounted our humiliations and crying as we vented our frustrations, but always looking forward to graduation and the careers we hoped would take shape thereafter. However, knowing that I would not do another student's story justice—I am not entirely sure I can do my story justice—I am sticking to my own.

I should also note that while this account by necessity dwells on my trials and tribulations, I fully recognize that I am extremely privileged, and that I have been blessed with an opportunity only available to a miniscule minority. The angst I occasionally express is certainly relative. I am not writing this story to elicit pity. I have witnessed real suffering, as all doctors do, and any sympathy experienced by the reader should be directed to the patients I am training to serve.

Moreover, these stories represent my reality during medical school; they will vary in significance and may not all be of equal interest. I do not want to give the impression that I endow every moment with cosmic significance. What I recount has been formative for me, but I do not imagine myself changing lives one recollection at a time. I have written this book for those who are curious about the often unpredictable and frequently unglamorous experiences of a third year medical student, and it pretends to be nothing more.

Finally, this book is a series of true stories, not a novel. However, characters' names have been changed in order to protect individuals' identities. These are the professions and disclosures of a standard memoir, but this particular book has an advantage that many memoirs do not: I am writing these stories as they happen, first as rough notes almost immediately after the occurrences, and then as full drafts a few weeks later. To be sure, this means that my perspective has an inherent naiveté, but it also means that the details are fresh and the integrity of my memory is uncontaminated. Who knows how these stories would be remembered and told several years hence?

I am inviting you to join me on my journey to fill a doctor's shoes (more likely than not, Dansko's), starting with my third year of medical school. The following stories reveal my failings, fears, embarrassments, and maybe even a few successes as I moved from the boards to the wards.

CHAPTER 1

Ugh, I don't know anymore, and I hardly even care… B, C, D. Everyone else in the exam center is leaving around me. A lady in combat boots (at least by the sounds of them) is stomping from computer to computer, wiping monitors and turning them off. A, C, D, B… I don't know, but I actually *do* care, so I frantically fill in my final answers as my eight-hour clock dwindles to zero. The exam program shuts off and all that is left on my computer monitor is, "Thank you for participating in the United States Medical Licensing Exam: Step One." Oh, you're welcome, and please, the pleasure was all mine. Right… I feel like I have been punched in the gut. The test that consumes a medical student's thoughts for the first two years of their curriculum just ended. While acceptance to medical school is challenging enough, the struggle doesn't end there. The opportunity to secure a spot in a great residency program after graduation depends on how we perform in medical school, with significant emphasis on our scores on this particular exam.

In theory, the nightmare was over. I had envisioned this moment for months. But for some reason, I did not sprint out of the exam center, pop a bottle of champagne in the parking lot, and sing at the top of my lungs. Instead, I slowly gathered my belongings (primarily the entire pizza that I brought for fear I would get hungry during the exam) and trudged to my car. I felt nauseous. Our career options rode on this test, and now it was over, and there was nothing I could do about it anymore. I felt helpless.

I started on my drive back home, and instead of immediately calling my family and friends to howl in celebration, I started crying, and didn't stop until the next day. Sure, I spoke to my family and friends in between tears, and I was sure to feign enthusiasm when they exclaimed, "You're all done! Can you believe it?" (Because let's be honest, I am sure they were equally relieved, if not more so, that they didn't have to hear about "The Defining Test of my Life" anymore). But I didn't feel excited. The stress of the previous two years decided to manifest itself as waterworks. I admit I am an emotional person, and oddly I hadn't cried much over the previous two years. Deep down, I knew I didn't have time to cry. Now, though, I had a week off until third year of school started, so I had plenty of time to drain both my brain and my tear ducts, and the tears just continued to flow.

Bit by bit, the tears slowed, and the weight on my shoulders lifted. In its place, relief settled in. I visited a friend in Miami for my vacation, and it didn't take much more than a frozen margarita (two at the most) before I was feeling like I thought I deserved to feel after completing my first and most important round of medical boards. It finally started to sink in that my classes and labs were over, and all I had left were clinical rotations. I was finally going to take all of the facts that I had learned from a textbook and apply them to a real, live person. It is the moment that all medical students wait for and the reason we go into medicine. It was springtime in Miami, the margaritas were flowing like water, and life was starting to look pretty good.

CHAPTER 2

Although the third year of medical school is a
confusing period for those who live through it, its
basic aim is simple enough: to provide students with
an opportunity to gain experience in all of the major
areas of medicine. My class of 160 students rotated
through internal medicine, neurology, psychiatry,
obstetrics/gynecology, orthopedics, family medicine,
surgery, emergency medicine and pediatrics. We all
go to different hospitals or clinics and work in all of
these fields at different times.

These individual rotations separated my life into
discrete segments, making any account of this period
more like a collection of short stories than one long
narrative. The fundamental objective of third year is
to learn how to care for patients, but students are also
constantly preoccupied with finding a specialty that
matches their interests and skill set. Apart from these
two common and broad goals, not much unifies the
rotations. On each one, we learned different
medicine, different procedures, and worked with
different types of people. It was a revolving door of
people, information, and tasks, but luckily I did have
one person looking out for me.

My "preceptor," or mentor, was the one continuous
support guiding me through my experiences and
through her I was able to find some continuity
during third year. All medical students are paired

with a doctor in their first year of medical school, and the partnership with your preceptor is a valuable constant in our often-tumultuous medical school career. In the first two years, we spend the vast majority of our time learning from books, but thanks to our preceptors, we receive some clinical experience working with a doctor during this time as well. My preceptor happened to be an emergency medicine physician, so for the first couple of years of school, I was convinced I would do emergency medicine. She was excellent and I wanted to be like her when I finally became a real grown-up doctor myself. For two years straight, I worked with her every couple of weeks, and would continue to do so for the rest of medical school. She was the only person who could observe my metamorphosis from the beginning of medical school to the end, so she served as a point of reference for my progress, and thus was a particularly helpful (and appreciated) resource in my education.

Sampling from the smorgasbord of specialties is designed to give students an idea of what area of medicine we would eventually like to go into. By the end of our third year, most of us will have decided on a specialty, or at least that is the goal. Then, during our fourth year, we can do "elective rotations," which allow us to re-visit an area of interest or delve further into a subfield of medicine before we apply for residency programs.

Throughout these rotations, we work with a variety of professionals: nurses, physical and occupational therapists, social workers, and physician assistants, but as medical students, the majority of our experience will be spent with residents and attending physicians. A resident doctor is an individual who has graduated from medical school (and so officially has the title "Dr."), but is still completing a residency program in his or her chosen field of medicine. Residency programs vary in length—they can be anywhere from three years for a primary-care field, like family medicine, to seven years for a more specialized area, like neurosurgery—but "resident doctor" means the same thing regardless of the area in which one works. Residents have the same responsibilities that a physician in their field has, but they have their work monitored by an attending physician, which brings us to our second definition.

Attending physicians are full-blown doctors (not that residents are half-blown) who have completed their residency and now work in their respective medical field. In any given medical setting, you can generally pick out an attending physician by searching the room for the person with the biggest smile. Attending physicians are at the point in their career when they feel competent and efficient; their schedules are generally lighter and they are finally making some money. Residents make money too, but given the number of hours they work, their salary works out to be approximately $12/hour. Tempting, right?

Now, please, don't everyone apply for medical school at once—they can't handle that type of volume. Actually, I wouldn't blame aspiring doctors if they put down this book right now, applied for a position at the nearest Sears, and lived out their days as a happy salesperson. They'll probably make about as much as doctors do during the first several years of their medical careers while working far fewer hours, and they'll also have their first choice of an ever-changing array of clothes, made all the more valuable in that they aren't stained with fecal matter, blood, vomit, and/or various other bodily fluids (more on that later).

But I digress. My first rotation was OB/GYN, and I was scared. Not only was I new to this whole "taking care of patients" thing, but also I had to start in a particularly intimidating field. All areas of medicine can be sensitive and personal, and thus each of them provides a medical novice with a perfect venue for embarrassment. However, as soon as genitalia become the focus of an exam, there is an immediate increase in opportunities to fulfill our awkward quota for the day (a quota that was, for the record, frequently surpassed by me and other students).

I was assigned to St. Joseph's Hospital close to downtown Denver for my rotation. This was good news. I heard the residents and doctors were very nice, and there was free food and parking involved—all music to a medical student's ears. In addition, I had spent time volunteering in the ER at St. Joseph's before medical school.

I took on this volunteer role after my initial rejection from medical school; it was my attempt to beef up my application and acquire more clinical experience for my second round of applications. Every day I volunteered there, I looked at all of the residents and physicians with burning curiosity and a touch of envy. I yearned to be one of them. I was crushed by my rejection, and would do anything to be accepted the next time around. And things get even cheesier and perhaps a little pathetic from here—when I volunteered, I would sit in the Starbucks outside of St. Joseph's and study for the MCAT so that I could occasionally glance up and see the doctors walk in with their white coats. It was my inspiration to keep working hard.

To many, this is pitiful, but doctors were as interesting to me as boy bands are to teenage girls, and I ached for them to talk to me. It all came full circle the first day of my OB/GYN rotation at St. Joseph's. One of the residents and I took a quick lunch break and decided to go grab coffee at that very same Starbucks. As we stood in line discussing the management of cervical dysplasia, I glanced over to a table on my right. There on the table was a Kaplan MCAT prep book. A girl was studying for the

Medical College Admissions Test, exactly as I had been doing three years ago! I looked down at my white coat—a very short white coat, to be sure, one designed to say "Warning: medical student only," but a white coat nonetheless—and back at her books. My heart felt as if it may actually burst from happiness and pride. This could have been a perfect coincidence, or maybe it was a sign with a message. In any case, I received a message loud and clear: I had finally made it. I was on the other side.

CHAPTER 3

The next couple of days went fairly well. The Starbucks episode still lingered pleasantly in the back of my mind. I walked lightly and I took on my tasks and responsibilities as an enthusiastic student beginning her third year of medical school. Naturally, these tasks and responsibilities were minor and included things like helping set up for surgeries, holding retractors for the surgeons, and "rounding on" patients at 5:30 in the morning.

Rounding for *doctors* refers to visiting patients who are staying in the hospital, checking the status of their health by completing a physical exam, ordering labs or studies that need to be done, and writing up a note based on the patient's progress. Rounding for *medical students* entails trying to see all of your patients before the resident does (who must see them before the attending doctor), which means 5:00 AM is typically our arrival time. After we check in with the nurses about overnight events, we awkwardly and intrusively wake up the patients by having to turn on lights, at times tripping over other sleeping family members, all the while apologizing and explaining we are medical students and that we must perform a physical exam. (As you might imagine, this isn't exactly a routine an ill person welcomes at the crack of dawn.) We then type up our "findings" into a progress note, which in theory should help the doctor do his or her job. What we are actually doing is taking our physical exam findings (which are very few at this stage in the game) and trying to type them up in a way that sounds like the textbooks we read in the first two years.

When you're rounding, normal English isn't sufficient anymore. Our notes must have an air of sophistication, even if the message can easily be conveyed without it. For example, we could no longer say something like "The rash is on the same side as her surgery — it looks like eczema and it doesn't seem infected." Instead we would write "The dermatitis is ipsilateral to her incision. It has features consistent with atopic dermatitis and there is no evidence of infection." If a patient describes the course of their symptoms in their own words, we must put them in quotes when we include them in our notes. We do this primarily to indicate that the language is the patient's, but it often seems like we want to distance ourselves from the patient's wording or phrasing, avoiding any use, however justified, of laymen terms. If we wrote, "The patient reports that the rash is 'itchy' and looks like 'little bumps,'" we would describe the itchiness as "pruritic" and the appearance of the rash as "papular." I've always found the way we deal with what patients say amusing; the quotations in our notes seem to suggest that we are skeptical of what they are saying, as if we don't believe the rash is actually irritating, and it only supposedly looks like little bumps.

To transform our language into medical speak is initially difficult, and it often takes us much longer to do than the resident or attending doctors. Soon after we think we have an acceptable note, the resident comes along, rounds on the same patients, and promptly undoes our note because often it is laden with medical student errors. As you can see, most of our work in the beginning consists of "playing doctor," which is exhausting for us and makes other people's jobs harder. Oddly enough, though, the residents and attending doctors are still up for teaching us. This might make their job more fun, but it definitely adds to their workload. I was very lucky to work with a great group of residents and attendings at St. Joseph's on my OB/GYN rotation. They didn't seem to mind the (not inconsequential) amount of teaching work I added to their daily routine.

Like most medical specialties, gynecology is best taught by giving students hands-on experience—by, say, letting us perform pelvic exams on patients who are under general anesthesia. A patient who is scheduled for a hysterectomy (uterus removal) or an oophorectomy (ovarian removal), for instance, is in need of general anesthesia, and once the patient is under, the surgeon always does a pelvic exam. Beforehand, students are encouraged to perform the same exam and report their findings. This allows the surgeon to follow their steps and then either affirm or correct the student's findings. The whole anesthesia component really provides the student with a sense of comfort; it enables a safe environment for the blushing and fumbling that would be noticed by a patient in a conscious state. Without the anesthesia, the situation isn't comfortable for anyone involved.

It was my turn for this opportunity, and I was to perform my first pelvic exam in the OR. The bright OR lights cast their characteristic fluorescent glow over the operating table where the woman lay, providing the type of illumination that makes everything appear sharper, even harsher, and the setting is made all the more dramatic by the chill of the OR. The room is kept cool for the surgeons because once sterile and gowned, they quickly become warm with the extra layers. Overtime, I grew to love the distinct burning glow and the uncomfortable chill of the OR.

While I had done a few pelvic exams before, I had never done one for an anesthetized patient, and I was excited that I could actually take my time and maximize a great learning experience. I apologize in advance for everyone with weak stomachs out there, but this is a tale about the trials and tribulations of becoming a doctor; I hope you didn't expect everything covered to be acceptable for discussion at the dinner table.

So there I was, two fingers in the patient's vaginal canal. Everything was going just fine. My attending stood beside me offering instruction and pointing out anatomical features that I should attempt to palpate. I was intensely focused on trying to feel the elusive ovaries[1] when suddenly I heard one of the residents to my left exclaim, "Oh, Emilee!! Wait, stop! She is-- Oh, no! Well, oh well." I looked up to see the look of horror/amusement on the resident's face. I followed her eyes down to my shoes. They were covered with suspicious excrement of sorts...Well, let's call a spade a spade: it was poop. I had put too much pressure on her rectum through her vaginal canal, causing the patient to have a bowel movement by no fault of her own...on my shoes. There are many situations, medical or otherwise, in which you are absolutely unsure how to proceed because you have never even imagined something like it. I can safely say that this was one of those times.

Do I laugh? Because let's be honest, there was clearly some humor in the situation. Do I cry? Because if we are being honest, I considered that option too. Should I vomit? In theory, things like this shouldn't bother me, but I was completely blind-

---

[1] *I don't think I ever successfully felt the ovaries, or any ovary for that matter.*

sided and ill-prepared to deal with such a surprise. Or do I play it cool? After all, I am trying to become a professional, and bodily excrement is pretty standard in the medical world. I decided on a combo: I chuckled (albeit uneasily), grimaced, and slowly backed away from the patient, professing my apologies to everyone in the room (and to my poor Dansko's, which were fortunately partially protected by the mandatory surgical paper booty). Fearing further damage, I slowly slid myself and my soiled shoes to the nearest trash can where I could proceed with the cleanup. Needless to say, they had me exit the OR and "re-scrub in" to ensure sterility for the proceeding operation, and luckily the remainder of the procedure went smoothly and cleanly.

CHAPTER 4

While this was an uncomfortable situation, it was at least comical. I can certainly see the humor in it now, and even had some appreciation for it at the time. However, I had another uncomfortable, but altogether different, experience soon after, one that I don't wish upon any medical student ever, let alone one in their very first clinical rotation. It was about a week later and I was still on my OB/GYN rotation. Every CU student does Labor and Delivery for two weeks (one week of day shifts, and one week of night shifts). The gods of OB/GYN seem to have an agreement that everything terrible will happen at night. This night was no different.

At the hospital, with her husband, was a woman in labor who had undergone IVF (in vitro fertilization) treatment in order to become pregnant. They were an older couple around 40, and this was their first pregnancy. The embryo implantation is the hardest component of IVF impregnation for an older couple. It is a tricky procedure to begin with, and the older a woman is, the more likely it is to fail. This couple was certainly on their fertility decline, so the fact that they became pregnant was certainly lucky, and their excitement was obvious.

Up until this point, I had not been involved in the direct care of this couple, but heard the residents talking about the situation. The woman had been laboring for hours, and was not progressing (dilation of the cervix had stopped). She was almost completely dilated, but not to the requisite 10 cm, which is necessary for a vaginal delivery. Obstetricians do what they can to promote vaginal deliveries because the benefits for both the baby and the mother far outweigh those of a cesarean section. The physicians and the couple were holding out for a natural vaginal delivery. Around 3:00 AM, one of the other residents went to check on her progress. Soon after, a robotic voice came over the hospital's loudspeaker: "Code C in room 210…Code C in room 210…" "Code C" is the signal for an emergency C-section, and are dreaded words on Labor and Delivery.

Back in the resident and nurse lounge, everyone sprang to life. I was sitting there studying for my upcoming exam and didn't know which end was up. Everyone around me filed out of the room within seconds and fled into the OR. It wasn't clear that I was invited, but I had scrubbed into several C-sections and knew sterile protocol, so I followed everyone in.

To be faced with an emergency situation is highly stressful, but this isn't news to anyone. Everyone can relate to the immediate adrenaline rush that accompanies this type of setting. The flushing of one's face, the instant racing of the heart, and the uncomfortable tacky feeling of your skin all represent

our body's way of saying "it's go time." These signs
of stress are particularly helpful if you have to run
from a bear (as we so often find ourselves having to
do), but when the situation demands that your brain
remain alert and sharp, these indicators of stress are
pesky and downright detrimental. So, over time a
physician must develop ways to appropriately deal
with, and essentially suppress, these interfering
symptoms. I had an emergency physician once
explain her tactics for overcoming stress. It was early
in my training and I inquired about her ability to
make serious, often complicated decisions while
faced with a medical emergency. She explained to
me, "Emilee, when you are confronted with a patient
in a life-threatening emergency, you have to
remember that this isn't *your* emergency. Remember,
you are healthy, safe, and at the end of this, you will
go home to your family." Initially I thought this
seemed crass and selfish, but then I realized the
importance of this attitude. In fact, it is this attitude,
and this attitude alone, that allows physicians to save
lives. They have to remain detached and levelheaded
regardless of the situation. This is the only way they
can continue to think clearly and help patients
during *their* time of emergency. To quote the classic
satirical novel *The House of God* (which I read before
medical school, but only now have a true
appreciation for): "During a cardiac arrest, the first
procedure is to take your own pulse." Indisputably,

this type of medical maturity takes years to master. While the other OB/GYN surgeons had more than likely achieved such enlightenment, I was nowhere near this state of mind when I was confronted with the crash C-section that night.

It was a sight to behold. The nurses came running in with the mother and she was wheeled quickly into the OR, hitting the door on the way in, an unfortunate but fitting way to convey the frantic nature of the situation. There were about 12 people fully gowned and masked in the room, bustling around. There were 3-4 people off to the side from the neonatal team ready to resuscitate the baby if needed. Several nurses made preparations as surgical technicians helped the surgeons gown and prepare for the operation. The anesthesiologist was organizing equipment in order to put the patient under general anesthesia—not typically used for a c-section, and not always used even in crash c-sections, but in some scenarios, including this one, it is the only thing quick enough in an emergency. According to the guidelines used for emergency C-sections, the baby should be out of the mother in less than twenty minutes of officially declaring that an emergent c-section is necessary. That includes all of the time it takes to coordinate the necessary staff members, as well as transporting the patient to the OR. By the time the patient has entered the OR, there are usually only minutes left before the baby needs to be out.

This timeframe includes putting the mother under general anesthesia, making the incision through the abdominal layers all the way through to the uterus, and grabbing the baby out. Under normal circumstances, it can take at least 5-10 minutes just to administer the anesthesia, and another 10 minutes or so is required for the abdominal incision.

I was standing in the room like a mannequin, but I was tucked away in a corner, so I knew I wasn't messing anything up too badly. I watched everyone dance around me, as if they were taking part in some ritual that I had not yet been initiated into (which is in fact close to being true). I continued to just stand there with lead shoes, scared for everyone in the room, but mostly for myself. In situations like these, med students so desperately want to be helpful, but don't know how to be, and in reality probably should just stand clear.

Soon the husband came in with a nurse. He took one look at the scene and the color drained from his face. As important as it is for spouses to be present (or at least be able to be present) at the birth of their child, an emergency C-section is absolutely not the place for them. It is messy, loud, and at times it looks barbaric. The care that patients receive is of course anything but barbaric, but it can certainly look that way.

One of the residents looked at me and asked, "Actually Emilee, can you please wait in the hallway with Mr. S?"

I quickly nodded. I had already learned that I should treat all questions as commands. As I smiled at him and walked out into the hall, my first reaction was *Wow, now this is an important job to ask of a medical student!* Then my second thought was, *Holy shit!!! Now THIS is an important job to ask of a medical student!*

What was I supposed to say or do with him? I took one look at the color of his face and then quickly searched around for a chair, preparing for what seemed like an inevitable faint. As I was doing so, I was verbalizing my thoughts out loud to break the silence. (That is, I mentioned I was looking for a chair, not that I thought he was going to faint.) He quickly assured me he didn't want to sit and started pacing.

Oh no, I thought, *he doesn't look so good.* What will I do if he hits the deck? I quickly started reviewing the ABC's of CPR in my head, and then stopped as quickly as I started. *No, you dummy. If he passes out, it is likely a vasovagal reaction due to his overactive sympathetic nervous system. It won't be a cardiac arrest. Duh.*

My thoughts continued to flounder. *Ok, what next?* I noticed he had an accent. *Should I ask him where he is from? Oh for heaven's sake. No! He is not in the mood for small talk. Should I try to explain the situation?* Again, I had been on OB/GYN for a mere two weeks and had only been a part of a few c-sections, so I wasn't confident that I could explain exactly what was going on. *Should I reassure him?* This is what I wanted to do, but I hadn't even met him or the mother, and more to the point, I wasn't sure of the situation. I didn't want to give false hope about something I knew nothing about. Essentially all I knew at this point was how important this pregnancy was to him and that it could potentially end disastrously, and I would likely be with the father when he first found out.

I always knew I would face difficult situations becoming a doctor. When we had our "delivering bad news" communication sessions, I knew it was important to pay attention, but I never imagined that I would have to implement anything I learned so soon, when I still felt so incompetent. Later, having given the matter a moment's thought, I realized that I would, of course, not be the one to deliver any bad news if there was any to report. The doctors would come out and take over, but anxiety can often cloud your perception of a situation or the role you are supposed to play in that situation.

My hesitation notwithstanding, I started to give reassurance anyway, although this was tough because I wasn't assured myself. The last thing I wanted to do was lie to the expectant father. I settled for saying really vague and generic things that were true, but don't necessarily carry a lot of weight:

Playing Doctor

"Don't worry, this happens all the time. They are great surgeons who...." I didn't have to worry about finishing because he cut me off and anxiously asked, "Can she feel that?!?"
From behind the OR doors were guttural cries from the mother. Normally, I would attempt to explain that this is totally normal. "She is just feeling pressure," I might say, "because she is under a spinal block, which blocks pain, but not all feeling, and so pressure remains."

However, I knew that in this case, the patient was supposed to be under general anesthesia, and not a spinal block, and so shouldn't feel anything. *Why was she screaming like that?* I decided to go with the spinal block and "pressure" sensation explanation anyways. I felt helpless and overwhelmed. Even if something had gone awry and she wasn't completely under yet, I certainly didn't want the father to know she was feeling everything. To this day, that might make me a liar, but at the time I felt like *I* was about to pass out. Between the father of the baby and I, it was a race to the floor. (I later found out that in some circumstances surgeons make the first cuts even if the anesthesiologist is still putting the patient under anesthesia. It is certainly not ideal, but in emergency situations it is necessary. And to be honest, the pain the mother experienced was probably not that much worse than the pain of a vaginal delivery, not that the latter is easy to endure. But having not gone through either of these, I can't be too sure.)

Then silence replaced her cries, and the ominous change blanketed the hallway. Though the quiet seemed almost worse, and I started to fumble with reassurance again. It didn't take long before I decided that as awkward as I felt with the silence in the hallway, I would just shut up. Neither of us knew what to say or how to act, so why pretend? Again, the whole procedure should happen exceptionally quickly, so while it felt like I spent my entire shift out there, it was actually only a matter of minutes before we heard the cry of the newborn. We looked at each other and smiled. What some people consider "the most annoying sound on earth" was at the time as beautiful as the opening movement in Tchaikovsky's 1812 Overture. He chanted, "Thank you Jesus! I will never ask for anything again! Thank you Jesus!"

I had just been a part of, arguably, the most important and stressful time of this man's life, and now was able to share in the best moment of his life. This was one of the most powerful connections I have ever experienced with another human.

Fortunately, everything turned out okay medically, but in a lot of ways, I felt I had failed in one of the first situations in which I could truly help. The entire time we are in medical school, and particularly in our third-year clinical rotations, we yearn to be helpful. While medical school is challenging in a number of ways, many of us struggle the most with feeling out of place. It's hard not to consider yourself a burden to the true professionals around us. We are constantly trying to skirt to the sidelines. We dodge people left and right in busy procedural rooms and often apologize in advance before asking questions, even though these questions are almost always warranted. We are constantly evaluating and criticizing ourselves as we struggle to make the residents' lives easier.

So, at long last, I was in a situation in which I could have been *genuinely* helpful, and I don't think I was. In hindsight, it is clear that I didn't need to know the specific details of the procedure behind the OR doors, nor did I need to explain all of the different possible outcomes of the operation. I only needed to know how to be a caring human, one ready to help another concerned, vulnerable human in whatever way I could. While many of us medical students pride ourselves on our ability to empathize and communicate with others (hence our chosen profession), our virtues are not always at our beck and call. When I stood in the hallway outside the OR room, I truly wasn't sure how to act. I lost myself. We are taught communication skills, but the vast majority of our training involves learning black and white answers. We are taught to memorize facts, learn procedures, and apply the advances of science to specific ailments. It was clear that my late night anatomy and pharmacology cram sessions weren't going to be bail me out of situations that called only for compassion.

When I confronted the "Code C," I had an all-or-nothing response. I wanted the concerned future father to hear only the words of an expert. As far as I was concerned, if I didn't say everything perfectly, I would fail, thereby heaping more stress on the shoulders of an already stressed man. Looking back, I now recognize that it hardly mattered what I said to him. He just needed support, even if it was silent support, and I didn't need to be a hero or expert to provide such a thing.

CHAPTER 5

By the time my OB/GYN rotation had ended, it was June, and summer was in full swing. Unfortunately for me, this didn't mean a whole lot. There aren't too many camping trips or barbeques for a third year medical student. My enthusiasm for medicine was renewed after my first rotation, though, and this was enough to propel me through some of the long summer days and partially alleviate my chronic fear that I was missing out on life.

Although I was acutely aware of my shortcomings during the OB/GYN rotation, the overall experience lingered pleasantly in my mind. I may have handled the expectant father less than perfectly, but the result of his wife's pregnancy was certainly a good one, and similar happy outcomes led me to start seriously considering it as a career choice. I was a part of many wonderful moments, like the first delivery I ever observed. After the baby was delivered and settled on the mother's chest, the OB/GYN began stitching the mother's vaginal laceration. She glanced up at me to explain the type of suture she was using, took one look at my face and broke into an ear-to-ear grin. My whole mask was fogged up from the condensation of my own tears—tears of incredulity and elation. I was emotionally overwhelmed by the experience.

I was also involved in a triplet c-section—so involved, in fact, that I technically named the babies! We knew the triplets would be girls, and the parents had already selected their names, but they wanted the surgeons to name them in whatever order they chose as they were delivered. The resident and attending tasked me with this joyfully surreal opportunity. The first baby came out and I excitedly announced, "Here is Stella!" A minute later, I exclaimed, "Meet Sonia!" Finally, as the last baby was delivered, I said, "This must be Sierra!" (These names have been changed for confidentiality, but the alliteration was the same, using a "P" instead.) To say I was heart warmed would be a gross understatement. These and similar experiences were amazing, but this was my first rotation, and I was only six weeks into my third year. I recognized that the novelty of being in the hospital was at least partially driving my enthusiasm. I knew I had a lot left to see.

Next up was my first preceptor shift of third year. It is usually regarded as an additional and somewhat inconvenient task we have to complete in the midst of finding enough time to study, but I felt excited for this particular shift. My first clinical rotation had made me feel more comfortable and competent with patients, and I looked forward to showing my preceptor the transformation that I was undergoing. Because the first couple of years are so classroom-and textbook-oriented, the initial time with these mentors feels awkward and foreign. No matter how personable a medical student may be, talking with patients about their personal health and performing physical exams feels intrusive when you are only used to interacting with human bodies in diagram form. It takes an immense amount of time and relentless repetition to feel comfortable with patients. The requisite level of comfort begins developing throughout our third and fourth year rotations, but won't be complete until well into residency.

Many students only report awkward *clinical* encounters while working with their preceptor, but I was able to demonstrate my incompetence in many more ways. One of my first preceptor shifts, which was early in my first year of school, can serve as an illustrative example, although I could cite plenty of others.

In this particular instance, I was nearing the end of my shift, so I thanked my preceptor and told her that I looked forward to seeing her next time. I wanted to end the shift on a good, fulsome note, and therefore wanted to avoid asking how to navigate out of the ER to the parking lot. It couldn't possibly be that hard, and I figured I would just walk around until I made my way out. In any field that requires personal expertise, the desire to keep one's pride intact is overwhelmingly, and frankly irrationally, strong. To a medical student, asking for help is uncomfortable, even if it is just on a simple matter like exiting a building. To me, asking for help was a bit like stopping a homeless guy to see if you can have a bite of his burrito—you just wouldn't do it, even if you really want to find the exit or the burrito looks particularly delicious. Looking back, this seems just as unreasonable as I am sure it seems to you now.

Of course, I had no idea what I was doing, and this became painfully clear when just moments after saying goodbye to her, I somehow ended up locked in a hallway, imprisoned by doors that both needed an official badge to exit. I had no such badge. *What kind of an obtuse operation was this?* I couldn't believe that a hallway had been designed in a way that let people in without a badge, but not back out. For a second I wondered if this was an intelligence test and glanced over my shoulder for a camera. I set my paranoid thoughts quickly aside, though, and decided to just wait it out. Someone would come through the hallway at some point, right? I had my preceptor's phone number, so technically I could have called for a rescue at any point, but I would have rather taken one of the doors off the hinges with my bare hands than admit to her that I managed to trap myself minutes after I had so breezily exited my shift.

Finally, after at least 10 minutes, someone did walk through the doors. I was playing it cool on my phone when the door opened. By "playing it cool," I mean "pretending that I received a really interesting email the second before I opened the door." But I was playing a dangerous game: the email had to be interesting enough to justify my bizarre reading location, a small hallway, but not so interesting that I didn't grab the open door the moment it opened, abandoning the email and breaking for freedom. No one seemed to notice anything strange, though. I suppose I *had* played it cool (as ironic as that seems in this particularly uncool situation). I reached the parking lot shortly after escaping captivity and drove off with my preceptor none the wiser.

After a mere two months, though, I managed to set myself up for embarrassment again, and this time my fall wouldn't be entirely private, like the hallway incident. I was just finishing up my shift with my preceptor and headed out to the parking lot. (I knew where it was at this point.) I climbed in my car and made my way to the exit gate. In all of my previous experiences, this gate was open at this time of evening, but not tonight, and it was clear I would have to pay to exit. Normally, this would be unfortunate, but not cause for panic. However, I didn't have the requisite cash for the machine, and in fact I didn't even have my wallet. I had forgotten to transfer it from my gym bag to my backpack earlier. *Crap! What was I supposed to do?*

I quickly scanned the area to examine what barriers I was up against—could I realistically and inconspicuously drive over any of them? (Typically, I consider myself an honest person, but when criminal behavior is pitted against looking foolish to your preceptor, criminality wins every time.) However, I drive a Honda sedan, so the dream of four-wheeling my way out of this mess was squelched as soon as the idea danced across my panicking neurons. For a brief moment, I even wondered how much damage my car would incur if I just drove straight through the wooden gate. Maybe a couple scratches here and there, but I didn't care that much about my car, and if I got caught maybe I could somehow claim it was an accident. Obviously, irrationality had taken hold. The fear of having to go back inside to ask my preceptor for money was clouding my judgment. I had one final thought before giving up, and that was to re-park my car and to do some good old-fashioned panhandling. After all, I was downtown at Denver Health. The neighboring intersections see plenty of beggars every day. Most people wouldn't bat an eye, and I only had to earn three dollars. Two things (and only two things) made this seem less than ideal: it was 11:00 PM, and I was wearing scrubs. It was clear that I was going to have to go back inside and admit that while I came prepared for work, I was not prepared to leave it. I walked around until I found my preceptor, and then had to ask to borrow money. Ouch. She was, as you might expect, understanding and gracious, and I guess I didn't adequately consider this possible reaction when I was considering driving my car through the gate.

Now that you understand some of my history with my preceptor, you may appreciate why I was now excited for my first shift with her during third year. I was excited at the opportunity to potentially perform more like a functioning clinician and less like a drunken bat.

As it turned out, my excitement was correctly placed. This particular shift was one of my more successful medical school experiences. Of course, a good portion of my success can be attributed to fortuitous coincidence—I had just finished my OB/GYN rotation, which was lucky given the patient I encountered. A 36-year-old woman presented to the emergency department with a day of vaginal bleeding and some left, lower abdominal pain. This is a presentation full of obstetrical and gynecologic implications, and so the one field of medicine in which I now had practical experience was directly applicable to the case before me. I actually stood a chance of understanding the patient's condition and might even know what to do about it. After talking with her and performing a physical exam, I returned to my preceptor to tell her about the patient. I explained everything that I had asked the woman, detailed the manner in which I had examined her, and recounted what I thought our next plans should be, including urine pregnancy test, a complete blood count, a pelvic exam, and a pelvic ultrasound. I explained that I was worried about an ectopic pregnancy, and given the serious nature of this condition, wanted to rule this out first and foremost. My preceptor was nodding her head and the corners of her mouth were turned down—not in a frown, but in a way that an expert does when a rookie impresses them. In a way that says "I remember when I had to tell you which end of the stethoscope to place on the patient, and now you have a reasonable diagnosis and plan for the patient. Not bad." If I had a tail, it would have been wagging. This whole doctoring thing wasn't so bad.

Happily, the patient did not have an ectopic pregnancy. Instead, it was likely that she had undiagnosed endometriosis (severe, out-of-the-ordinary pain most often associated with the menstrual cycle), and we referred her to a primary care physician for follow up and further care. At this point, I wasn't worried that I incorrectly diagnosed the patient. I had outlined an evaluation and a plan that a physician would have done. For now, that was enough for me.

CHAPTER 6

During the first two years of medical school, and in fact before I even began my program, I heard heartwarming stories of the bonds that develop between medical students and their patients. Whenever I heard of these touching connections, I imagined what such an experience would feel like. I pictured myself sitting at a patient's bedside chatting about life and our common interests, soaking up their infinite life wisdom for hours on end and days at a time. With this idyllic image in mind, my first meaningful relationship with a patient took me by surprise. The first connection I felt with a patient was on my neurology rotation and none of the features that I thought were important to building a bond were a part of our relationship.

His name was M.M. (or at least that's what I will call him here for confidentiality reasons). He was an 83-year-old gentleman staying on our service because he had suffered an inferior cerebellar stroke, at the base of his brain. A stroke that affects this area and the surrounding nerves can affect your ability to balance, swallow on your own, and speak—one's voice can become very hoarse (almost non-existent) after this type of stroke. M.M. suffered from all of these symptoms, making it fairly clear he had had an inferior cerebellar stroke. And on top of the recent stroke, he had baseline Alzheimer's, so his cognitive abilities were already hindered before the stroke.

M.M. presented during the first week of my neurology rotation, and was sent from the ER up to the neurology service. I was with a couple of other medical students in this division of the hospital, and we took turns taking the patients that came to our neurology service. My resident looked at me and said, "are you ready? You're up for the next patient." I nodded as enthusiastically as possible, as any standard brown-nosing medical student does, and listened as the resident gave the patient's history and his current presentation. I was mentally groaning to myself, *Ugh, I don't want some old guy with Alzheimer's and a new stroke. This is going to be impossible.*

My job was to go see the patient and perform a thorough neuro exam so that later in the morning I would be prepared to present the patient to our attending physician. These are pretty standard expectations, so I set off to the neuro ward without too much apprehension, mentally reviewing the neuro exam in my head as I walked.

I entered the room and immediately stopped in my tracks. I backed out into the hallway to check the room number, convinced I had wandered into the wrong place. As it turns out, I was exactly where I was supposed to be: there was M.M., circus performer extraordinaire, at least from the looks of it. He had his bed completely folded and he was in the middle of it. Both the top and bottom halves were elevated as far as they went, forming a "U" shape. His body was correctly positioned on the bed, with his head and feet at their proper ends, but his face was close to his knees and he was flailing about. I looked around for the nurse (a common reaction when I am lost and need help), who happened to be outside his room. She just chuckled when she saw my face and explained that they had been trying to flatten the bed out, but he kept returning it to that position. I thanked the nurse for the information and turned to face my new patient. *What is this? Am I expected to talk to him and perform a neuro exam? Where is the 20-week pregnant lady that I can do an ultrasound on?* I wanted to run back to the resident's lounge and tell them I didn't want this patient, that it was too complicated and that I would never be able to perform an exam. I slowly approached the bed, calling out his name to verify I was with the right patient, and then prepared to introduce myself as the medical student who would be helping take care of him.

Unlike most stroke victims, he was a spry little thing, and as I introduced myself, I barely heard him whisper, "That's a pretty name." At first, I thought, *oh no, not again.* I had just come from a rotation at the Veteran Affairs Hospital and had plenty of winks from old men to last for the rest of my life. However, this comment left a lasting impression on me: those were the last words (besides his own name) I ever understood him say to me. His stroke had severely affected his voice; it was so hoarse that you could not make out what he was even *attempting* to say.

I explained that I was going to do a neuro exam, and proceeded to try to flatten out his bed. As I did so, he continued to thrash around, making an exam almost impossible. Only later did I learn that a patient's position in their bed is an excellent indicator of their level of agitation. The zanier the position, the more agitated the patient is likely to be. Given that M.M., suffering from Alzheimer's to begin with, had just had a stroke, and was in a completely foreign environment, he was understandably delirious and agitated, and he was clearly expressing this with his body language. I did the best I could with the exam, bid *adieu* to M.M. for the day, and then returned to the resident's lounge, where I prepared my presentation to be used when we rounded on him later. I was still feeling annoyed that I had him for a patient while other medical students had "interesting cases" — a guy with Guillain-Barre disease (a usually reversible paralysis that starts in the body's periphery and moves centrally after having a viral illness), a woman with isolated finger agnosia[2] (inability to recognize one's own fingers after a stroke), and another patient with transient global

---

[2] *I have never been, nor will I ever be, smart enough to understand the neurophysiology behind this.*

amnesia (complete loss of all memory for 24 hours). These are all textbook, classic patients that most medical students would be thrilled to help care for. Selfishly, I felt slighted by M.M.'s case.

At first thought, M.M. might seem as interesting as these other cases, and while his symptoms were classic for a cerebellar stroke, his neurologic exam and subsequent plan of care was muddled by the fact that he suffered from Alzheimer's at baseline. Like I explained, he was so delirious, and thus uncooperative, that it made his care seem annoying and too complex for me. The cases that the other students had weren't complicated by comorbid conditions, and on top of that, they were all very rare. The neurologists were practically salivating over them. (I don't mean this to be crude or make light of these conditions. This is a way in medicine to explain how interesting the science can be behind a disease. Don't worry, patients always receive the same level of care, regardless of how interesting a doctor deems their pathology.)

However, this was before I realized how close I would grow to M.M. He would remain my patient for the remaining month I spent on my neurology rotation. Every day I had something new and funny to report about him. Often it involved his mentally altered hospital roommate, who was also a brain injury patient. As odd as it sounds, M.M. soon became a part of my own identity on the rotation; the people I worked with couldn't help but associate him with me. The other students, residents, and attendings would look forward to my stories — "my adventures with M.M.," as everyone started fondly calling them.

Every morning I would greet M.M. and ask him for his name, his current location, and the year. The only thing I could ever understand was his name. Some mornings, he was so somnolent that I couldn't even get that minimal information out of him. When I could decipher his name, this was a good day. The entire time I was trying to talk to M.M., his "next door neighbor" would try to "talk" to me. I was never sure what his diagnosis was, but I always had to pull the curtain between his bed and M.M.'s to cut down on the distraction. While I was trying to extract basic information from M.M., the other patient would be yelling in a monotone voice, "heeeey laaady…. heeeeeyyyyyyy laaaadddyyy!!!!!" I had a hard time not laughing every time I went in to the room. After several attempts to get my attention, he would usually move on to ask for something to drink, and then when no one responded, he would engage in a cursing fit, talking about the incompetence of everyone in the hospital.

I rolled my eyes at M.M. Of course he didn't respond, but I felt like there was a part of him who understood.

Some days the neighbor was more cooperative. As part of M.M.'s neuro exam, I would have him follow commands. Usually they were things like "stick out your tongue" or "squeeze my fingers."

One day, I was talking to M.M. and asked him to stick out his tongue. The next door neighbor yelled aggressively, "What the hell for?" I chuckled to myself, and repeated the command to M.M. because he wasn't doing it. Again, "Hey M, stick out your tongue." Immediately from next door, "I am, dammit!!!"

This time, I laughed out loud and looked at M.M. for his response. I would like to think that I saw a twinkle in his eye, but it is possible that such a subtle sign was just my imagination.

The next day I came in and his neighbor was asking to borrow money (through the curtain, mind you). "Hey, can you lend me $50 bucks?? I swear I will pay you back." When he didn't receive a response from me, he revised his request "Okay, fine—how about $100??" M.M.'s situation, coupled with his (how should I put it?) colorful neighbor, made every morning in the hospital entertaining.

Unfortunately, given the nature of M.M.'s condition, his hospital course quickly became complicated. Because of his inability to swallow properly, he aspirated on his own saliva, causing pneumonia. On several of the mornings I visited, he could barely breathe. His lungs sounded like they were filled with water, as if he had gone snorkeling and didn't realize the top of the tube must stay above the water. He was somnolent most mornings and couldn't respond to my commands; his infection was progressing, which caused him to be delirious and agitated.

We started him on antibiotics, but this did little to quell the medical team's concerns about his well-being. Conversations commenced about the goals of M.M.'s care, and we discussed what the next appropriate clinical steps would be. (I say "we" discussed this matter, but for obvious reasons my contributions were limited, and by "limited" I mean "nonexistent.") Should we place a feeding tube? This is a very invasive procedure, but he was not eating on his own and could not tolerate anything orally because of his risk for continued aspiration. Should we discontinue his seemingly futile antibiotics? Sometimes elderly patient's elect for no antibiotic treatment as part of their "do not resuscitate" orders—his medical chart had gaps when it came to these legal details. Should we send him to hospice for comfort care only (measures that would control pain, but not prolong life)? It became clear that we needed to involve the family about their expectations of care and their desires for M.M., based on what his wishes would have been.

A couple days went by during which we continued to give him antibiotics and other supportive care.

Every day at rounds, we would deliberate over his care, trying to decide what would ultimately be best for him.

One morning, I went in for my regular visit and after I spent a few minutes with him, I was elated. M.M. was suddenly performing actions that just two mornings ago seemed impossible. He was able to say his first *and* last name for me, and even followed several commands with enthusiasm. He stuck out his tongue, and energetically raised his limbs in the air to touch my hands. What sounds like nothing to a healthy individual was great progress for M.M., at least as far as I could tell.

At rounds that day, I excitedly gave my report about M.M.'s improving condition and related the rest of my physical exam findings. I assessed and explained M.M.'s progress optimistically, and as I was concluding my presentation, I suggested that maybe we didn't need to pursue hospice care just yet.

A senior medicine resident was on our team, doing a neurology rotation for the month. She looked at me and solemnly related, "Emilee, you know that M.M. is going to die, right?"

My heart sank. I must have looked as crestfallen as I felt because she hurriedly followed up with, "I mean, I know it is disappointing, and that he has made small progress today, but he continues to wax and wane, and I have seen this hundreds of times.

Older patients like this, with this particular clinical picture, just don't do well."

I wasn't fooling anyone, but I tried to make up for my obvious disappointment by acting cool and detached, insincerely saying, "Yes, of course...I know...that makes sense..."

The group talked for a few more minutes about what would come next: arranging a family meeting and organizing hospice care. Everything they said seemed vague and distant while I tried to collect my thoughts.

I couldn't believe how discouraged I felt. Here was this elderly patient—a patient, you'll recall, who I didn't even want to follow at first because I was annoyed by his convoluted condition—who was pushing me to the verge of tears as I contemplated his quickly evaporating life. He couldn't even talk to me, and more likely than not he didn't even know who I was from day to day. However, at this point, I had seen him every day for almost four weeks, and somehow we had made a connection for reasons that still aren't entirely clear.

We spent the next several days contacting family members and arranging a meeting to figure out the ultimate goals of his care. Would they want a feeding tube placed? While this could provide temporary means of nourishment, is he an individual who would want this intervention? Did they want him in a hospice facility, or was there enough care and support for him at home? These and similar questions would soon need to be confronted.

After some deliberation, we finally settled on a time that would work for his two sons, two daughters, and a couple of his granddaughters. The resident asked me if I would like to start out the meeting, given that I knew M.M. the best out of the whole care team.

I was as honored as I was nervous. My first family meeting… I would have to explain what exactly had happened to M.M., why his hospital course was the way it was, why he wasn't improving, his probable prognosis, and what the options were from here. I wasn't thrilled by the idea, but knew that communicating with families is an important skill to practice. The resident physician assured me that she would be with me and could take over at any time. With this safety net in place, I agreed to the plan.

The morning of the family meeting, I went to see M.M., predicting it would be the last time I saw him. I knew the likelihood of the family wanting to place a feeding tube would be low because these are invasive, they dampen quality of life, and they do not significantly prolong life. With this in mind, I knew he would most likely be transferred to a hospice or home later that day. I walked into his room just as I had done over a dozen times before, and there he was, sitting up in bed wearing his glasses. It was the first time I had ever seen glasses on him. To me, it

was like he was in the middle of his daily routine—
just so normal—and I felt a familiar optimism,
similar to when he was able to follow my simple
neurologic commands. It was almost as if I had
walked in on him reading the New York Times and
enjoying a cup of coffee. Once again, I felt
encouraged, but it turns out that my optimism was
premature. His breathing was still so labored that I
didn't have to place a stethoscope on him to hear the
fluid in his lungs, and he was still temporally and
spatially disoriented. I knew the doctors were right.
Given his history of Alzheimer's, the severity of the
stroke he suffered, and the rampant pneumonia he
was now fighting, he would never be the M.M. that
people knew before this hospital admission.

I went through the normal routine with him, and at
the end, like always, I said, "hang in there Mr. M; we
are going to take care of you." At first I felt like I was
lying, and felt slightly shameful for it, but after more
thought I realized it wasn't a lie—we were still doing
just that. We were going to consult with his family to
figure out exactly the type of care M.M would want.
Maybe we could no longer care for his physical body,
but we could still provide care for his spirit by
acknowledging his wishes and intentions.

I walked down the hallway to the family meeting,
which was held in a small conference room on the 9th
floor of the hospital, amidst the patient rooms.
Anxiety pulsated through my body, and I could feel

the familiar (but unwelcome) lump start to rise in my throat at this rather inconvenient time.

In medical school, we often have conversations about crying with patients. We discuss first of all whether or not it is appropriate, and we also grapple with more specific questions, like when and with whom it's okay to cry. The general consensus is that it is okay to cry; however, you should cry only with the patients who you know well. Thus, someone like an E.R. doctor may not have many occasions to cry, or at least not in a professional context. Moreover, it's probably not a good idea to start crying before your patient does, and no matter what, you definitely shouldn't cry harder than your patient does.

Well, with the rate at which my throat was thickening on my way to the family meeting, I knew I was about to violate at least one of these guidelines, and so I took a minute to compose myself. I went to the restroom for a few minutes to think. I looked at myself in the mirror and was immediately glad I took the detour. I was clearly not in the best shape and my insecurities were readily apparent. I silently cursed my overactive autonomic system as red splotches started to creep up my neck. This was never going to work. I took a cold paper towel and began patting myself down, all the while giving myself a pep talk, mentally rehearsing the lines I was going to say. After a few minutes of this, I felt better and more in control, so I left the restroom, grabbing a quick drink of water on the way out. My resident was waiting for me outside of the room.

"You ready?" she asked as she smiled at me encouragingly.

"Yeah, I think I am," I replied, trying as best as I could to convince myself this was true.

Luckily, I had already met most of his family members. They had been supportive throughout his stay and were sometimes with M.M. in the mornings when I saw him.

I sat down and began my rehearsed speech. Everything went surprisingly smoothly. I covered what needed to be covered and then finished by explaining the possible courses of actions we could take with M.M.'s care. I took a deep breath and asked if there were any questions about anything I had said. The questions flowed in and I quickly looked to the resident for assistance. She took over. As she spoke, I felt relatively relieved about the way things went. Miraculously, I had managed not to cry at all. (Sometimes I cry just when I get nervous, even if I am not sad, so I had very low expectations for myself.)

The resident was explaining that because of his stroke, M.M. can't swallow and therefore can't eat for himself. The main question was whether or not we should place a feeding tube. We could also provide other, less-extreme comfort measures. We could continue antibiotics to keep the infection at bay (or at least at a dull roar) and alleviate some symptoms of his pneumonia. Or we could simply treat his pain. She continued to explain that due to his inability to swallow, he is prone to pneumonia (as we saw during this hospital stay), and thus even if he recovered fully from this one, it would only be a matter of time before he had another infection.

One of the daughters asked, "How long do you think he has if we placed a feeding tube?"

The resident responded, "It's really hard to know, but most likely a matter of months."

Science can predict and explain many things: the time it will take the earth to rotate around the sun, the progression of life from a single celled amoeba to a *Homo sapiens*, and how antibiotics can cure an infection, but science poorly predicts the life expectances of various illnesses. If forced to specify a time frame, physicians consistently overestimate the time an individual has left, and this inevitably leads to surprise and heartbreak for loved ones. Therefore, as a general rule, medical students are taught to predict remaining life using very general time frames (i.e. hours, days, weeks, months, years).

The daughter followed up with, "And what about without?"

"I don't know, maybe weeks to a month?"

At this point, one of the granddaughters, who couldn't have been older than eight, and therefore hadn't said anything up until this point, let out a little yelp, and then burst into tears.

It turns out I had congratulated myself too early. This was too much for me. I felt my eyes well up and soon spill over. Soon, the other adult daughters began to cry, and a relatively composed meeting quickly turned into an emotional one. I was starting to feel guilty, like I was causing their sorrow. However, luckily, right then, one of the daughters looked at me and mouthed "thank you," and I knew this was one of those times we discussed in school when it was okay to show emotion.

We talked a bit longer, and the whole family decided M.M. would never want a feeding tube. They would take him home, where they could take shifts caring for him 24 hours a day until his time eventually came.

On the way out, I felt obligated to say something else to the family. The best I could come up with was, "M.M. seemed like a great guy, and it was a pleasure to care for him."

One of the daughters teared up again and responded, "Thank you for all of your care. I know my father appreciated you every day when you came in."

While I knew there was no way anyone could really know that, given his non-verbal state, it was enough to put a smile back on my face for the rest of the day. In fact, I still smile about it. And I still reflect on it.

Initially, I felt deprived that I was assigned to M.M. I felt like I was truly at a disadvantage when compared to my peers and their "interesting" patients. But ultimately, I don't recall the other students building the same caliber of bond that I felt with M.M.

To this day, when I go see patients, I am still sometimes inclined to make a snap judgment about them or their diagnosis, but then I remind myself that I am capable of adjusting my perceptions. Those "less than ideal" circumstances may be a figment of my own attitude. Even if a relationship is difficult to establish, I am ultimately in charge of the connections I make with patients, and all of them have the potential to become another M.M.

CHAPTER 7

I used to think that all doctors were created equal. Before medical school and during the application process, I revered their success, admired their compassion, and envied their expertise. While the vast majority of physicians still embody these characteristics, there are some that have genuinely disappointed me. Initially, it was upsetting to meet them, and it was almost like the Christmas Eve when my uncle asked me if my brother still believed in Santa Claus. At the time, I still believed in Santa. After encountering a few less-than-excellent doctors, I worried that my perception of the profession might be nothing more than naïve idealism.

During the summer of my third year, I had a two-week orthopedic rotation. Orthopedics is an area of medicine that is not emphasized in the coursework portion of the program, even though it is particularly important for physicians to know. Any primary care physician or emergency doctor should know the anatomy of the musculoskeletal system in order to properly diagnose and treat injuries involving this system. For this reason, I was looking forward to those two weeks, as it might be one of the only opportunities I had to solidify my knowledge of this area before graduation.

Most of the rotation went smoothly, but on my last day, I was paired with a specialized orthopedic surgeon. He was nice enough to me, but the way he interacted with his patients was almost painful to watch sometimes.

To begin with, when the surgeon introduced himself to all of his new patients, he made sure to include his residency training program. Because it is such a highly regarded program in the medical community, it is obvious to me why he included it, but where he did his training is of no relevance to his patients, as virtually none of them will have any understanding of the relative merits of residency programs. His institutional namedropping, combined with other irritating habits of self-promotion, made his showmanship so grand that I had a hard time not laughing when he was speaking with a patient. The Orthopod was a parody of an orthopedic surgeon, going out of his way to bolster the arrogant stereotype that the nice orthopedists try so hard to combat.

One of the first patients of the day was a gentleman who had undergone a foot surgery for Charcot joint disease. This condition results from progressive peripheral neuropathy, which entails the gradual degeneration of nerves and eventually the destruction of a joint. These patients often need multiple operations and occasionally even amputations. Not only did this patient have a devastating disease that was severely affecting his quality of life, his surgery did not go as planned—the operation hadn't restored function to his foot (and we were there to break the news that we were at the end of treatment options). As much as I would like to take this as evidence of The Orthopod's technical incompetence (a kind of just recompenses for his lack of emotional intelligence), unfortunate things happen like this all the time in medicine, and even the best surgeons experience their fair share of bad outcomes.

Without giving too much thought to the ramifications this could have on the patient's life, The Orthopod flippantly explained, "Yeah, this sucks, but it happens. Unfortunately, there is not much we can do about it. You know, we tried…"

Naturally the patient was disappointed by this news, but he displayed a general sense of understanding as the conversation continued.

After a bit more discussion, he continued to explain, "Yeah, you have a progressive neuropathy. First it is your right foot, like it is now, but then it moves to your left foot, and then to your hands, and before you know it, you're screwed. You know?"

My heart was in my throat waiting for the patient's reaction. His face turned solemn and he nodded sadly. I couldn't believe how the conversation unfolded. While Charcot foot disease is often the result of poorly controlled diabetes, which is usually caused by the patient's poor lifestyle habits, this particular patient's neuropathy had nothing to do with his lifestyle. While I would have considered The

Orthopod's attitude terse and unjustified even if this patient *had* diabetes, it was especially inappropriate given that his nerve damage was simply poor luck. I felt nauseated and, as usual, helpless.

The patient remained very quiet, so The Orthopod quickly finished the conversation. After saying their goodbyes, I went to open the door for the patient. He was using a scooter for mobility, one in which you place your bad leg on a platform and use your good leg to scoot along. As I stood by the door, he wheeled past me and looked in my eyes and said, "Well, party on."

My heart ached, and frankly I was embarrassed. I wanted to run after him down the hall and say, "Please, come back. We can talk more about this if you want. I am sorry; I had nothing to do with this." Unfortunately, though, a rigid hierarchy exists in medicine, and to do this would so blatantly step on The Orthopod's toes that I didn't actually consider doing any of this. Self-preserving? Yes. Cowardly? Possibly. Unusual? No. I was there to keep the peace, work cordially with the surgeon, and pass the rotation.

Instead, all I could gather was, "Nice to meet you. Take care." As I watched him wheel down the hall and out of the clinic, I resolved to try and let this interaction slide. I gave the physician the benefit of the doubt, and convinced myself that this particular interaction was just a fluke.

But as he continued with his grandiose introductions and blunt, hurried explanations, I knew my initial disappointment with his first patient meeting was justified. My disappointment grew as the day dragged on, and I remember feeling especially disturbed after an appointment that came near the end of my time with him.

We saw a mother and her 19-year-old son who had broken his foot. The actual injury happened almost a year ago, and they tried to tough it out. The problem was that this family didn't have many resources. It was clear that they lacked money for both insurance and self-pay visits. Unfortunately, the foot's function had become so bad that despite their economic situation, they came to the clinic for evaluation. The mother was explaining that lately her son had not been able to perform his work (he was a house painter), and she was clearly expressing remorse at her decision to wait so long.

The Orthopod confirmed her fears, and then added to them. "Due to the nature of this fracture and the time that has elapsed, surgery may help, but it will likely have minimal benefit. It is quite possible that his career will be affected by his injury. Jobs that require long periods of standing or walking will not be feasible."

The mother sadly and regretfully responded, "but he is so young…"

Playing Doctor

Without skipping a beat, he replied, "well, that's obviously why you have to get insurance and keep insurance."

Well, I'll be damned… It's really just as simple as that? And all this time 50 million Americans were uninsured simply because they hadn't thought of that? This is revolutionary.

The Orthopod continued to talk about the details of the surgery. As he talked, I noticed a tear slip down the mother's cheek. I could tell that she was silently berating herself for letting this problem go untreated. Personally, I didn't think this made her a bad mother. She didn't know medicine well enough to know the ramifications, and she didn't have the resources to play it safe. There are currently thousands, if not millions, of Americans in her position.

It was like The Orthopod was unaware of anything he was saying. He finished up the meeting, said his goodbyes, and left the mother to consider whether or not they would schedule the surgery.

Again, I felt every muscle cell in my heart pulling. I desperately wanted to stay in the room and finish the conversation. Don't get me wrong; I know that it is as important for a physician to be direct with patients as it is to be a friend to them. As hard as it is, the reality of the situation must be delivered, regardless of how difficult the news might be to explain. Additionally, I realize I am still a novice at all of this. However, my point is a simple one: this doctor-patient consultation could have been done in a more sensitive manner.

This time, I didn't have the heart to leave without another word. I stopped at the door, squeezed the mother's shoulder and asked quietly underneath my breath if she was okay, shamefully trying to avoid the attention of The Orthopod who had already left.

Out of habit, she quickly mustered a smile and said, "yes." I knew that was unlikely, but again I was too afraid to stay. I quickly slipped out of the room to catch up with The Orthopod before we went into the next patient's room. This time, I felt like a coward through and through, but I also knew why I continued to go through the motions. My grade depended on pleasing the physician. In general, grades are very subjective during our third year, and a large portion of them is determined by whether or not the supervising physician likes you. On my last day of the rotation, I didn't feel comfortable risking my grade.

In the next patient's room, I was trying to think of excuses for why I had to leave early that day. Was I feeling a headache coming on? Maybe I had a little bit of a fever?

I didn't leave early. I carried on until the end of the day, but I felt let down and disenchanted with the medical profession. I also thought that perhaps I was crazy, and that all this time I had an unrealistically romantic view of doctors. Maybe this is what happens over time, and I, too, will be like this someday.

However, throughout the remainder of the day, an oath that all physicians take as medical students reverberated in my mind. It's called "the physician's oath" and it is deeply rooted in the medical tradition. It incorporates the infamous Hippocratic Oath, the one in which we all solemnly swear that as physicians we will "do no harm." It refers to the fact that medicine is as much an art as it is a science, often with no black-and-white answers. When we are unsure how to proceed with a patient, we must at the very least "do no harm." It sounds obvious, but in reality it takes immense practice, and that is why our training is so extensive. In theory, this oath should apply to all clinical situations, even though there are obviously some circumstances in which its application is more readily apparent. While The Orthopod is an excellent surgeon and will go to great lengths to "do no harm" in the OR, it seems he has lost his ability to apply the oath in all settings. Arguably, his clinical interactions were harmful. He left patients feeling defeated, guilty, or hopeless, and sometimes all three at once.

Initially, I felt frustrated that I had been paired with The Orthopod, and thought that I would never learn anything from his poor bedside manner. The truth is that I learn just as much from the bad doctors as I do from the good ones. I learn exactly what *not* to do and in a strange way it actually inspires me. I now know the impact that a doctor's words can have on a patient, even if what is said seems insignificant. If you can ruin someone's day in three seconds, you can improve it in an equally short amount of time.

I felt betrayed by someone who was meant to be a role model. Fortunately, I have met plenty of physicians who exemplify the professional I want to become and the person the public would be pleased to call their doctor. The orthopedist I worked with proved to be rare. These doctors exist, but they could not justifiably be called typical. Far more often, I feel inspired and rejuvenated by the physicians I work with, and when third year becomes tough, this is what fuels my motivation.

CHAPTER 8

Fourth of July came and went. As a child, this event always provoked anxiety for me. The holiday signified that summer was half over, and within a few weeks "Back to School" sales would be splashed all over town. Luckily, and unluckily, this day currently had little meaning to me as a medical student. I just finished the musculoskeletal rotation, and I had an entire new rotation to get through before I had a vacation, a break that was quickly morphing from "well-deserved" to "critical for my mental health." Ironically, it was indeed my psychiatry rotation.

I was scheduled to fulfill this requirement at The Children's Hospital. While there were both in-patient and out-patient programs there, I would primarily be working with children and adolescents in the in-patient setting.

I didn't know what to expect. The psychiatry portion of our curriculum primarily focuses on adult mental health. As a result, I felt ill-prepared to confront pediatric psychiatric pathology head on. However, I was very keen to learn more, and in fact I initially applied to medical school with the idea that I would become a psychiatrist. Since then, my early experiences with my preceptor began to steer me more towards emergency medicine, and my OB/GYN rotation had me seriously considering women's care for a career. Nevertheless, my strong initial interest in psychiatry kept my mind open to it.

On the first morning, I met the resident and the attending physician that I would work with for the month. They both seemed pleasant, and I was excited at the prospect of working with only two people. The attending physician began my tour around the facility, which seemed less about orienting me and more about explaining how to maintain the security of the building. We walked from the physicians' offices down the hallways to the children's in-patient rooms and treatment classrooms. There was a series of secured double door systems. In this case, "double doors" had two meanings: the classic one, in which every doorframe had two doors, but also two doorframes in a row, creating a double barricade system. I was strongly advised to wait for the closing "click" of one set of doors behind me before proceeding to the next set, and I was also instructed to approach the doorways walking backwards when I exited back through the doors, in order to avoid turning my back to any patients that could be loitering nearby, hoping for an opportunity to escape. Naturally, these are somewhat unnerving guidelines, but I expected to hear them ahead of time.

But then the instructions continued. I was showed the conference rooms where I would talk with patients. I was told to make sure that I never sat between the door and the patient because this might intimidate them, creating unwelcome aggression. At the same time, though, I was to make sure that I was at least equidistant between the patient and the door, and to never allow the patient between the door and myself. This was in case said aggression transpired, and in which case I would need a convenient escape route.

We continued on to the patients' rooms where the security was even more involved. Over time, things had become stricter and stricter, and there were lots of people working in this area to enforce the rules. I won't bore you with all the details, but there is one rule worth relating because I found it so unusual and troubling. It was a new rule, and it outlined bathroom expectations. When children went into their bathroom, they had to talk out loud the entire time they were in there. They were also supposed to hand over their scrubs (their uniform) to their respective "guard." Within the last couple of months, a young boy had successfully committed suicide by hanging himself on the shower bar by his scrubs.

As we finished up our tour, I felt anxious about the rotation. Mistakenly, I had pictured kids with general anxiety and behavioral conduct disorders, but the tour assured me I would be working with far sicker children.

Interestingly, for the first week of my rotation, it turned out that my apprehension was largely unwarranted. I was working primarily with run-of-the-mill rebellious teenagers and children with anxiety as a product of their disorganized home lives.

Then I met "Sophie." Sophie was a 14-year-old girl with what seemed like a typical story. She was admitted because the police had found her early that morning, a couple of miles from her house. Upon being caught, she threatened to hurt herself if they took her home (a very common threat in a runaway adolescent), so she was taken to the ER, and finally admitted to us for psychiatric evaluation.

The attending and I did the first couple of interviews together to hear her story. We both introduced ourselves and the psychiatrist started the interview. I assumed we would hear a story about how her parents wouldn't let her hang out with a particular friend, so she ran away. I was wrong.

"So Sophie, tell us, what happened today?" the psychiatrist began.

"I was trying to run away from home, but I accidentally went the wrong way, and ended up by my school instead."

"And this is where the police found you?"

"Yes."

"I am curious. Why were you running away from home?"

"My friend Red needed my help."

"Why does this friend need help?"

She nonchalantly carried on, "Oh, because Red is about to undergo an apocalyptic transformation."

This was getting interesting.

The psychiatrist pressed on but dodged the obvious for now, "Oh okay. So Red, is this friend a boy or girl?"

"Boy."

"How did you meet him?"

"On the internet."

"Where does he live?"

"In England."

"Oh wow, so very far away. Is he visiting the United States?"

"No, I was going to Florida to meet him, so he could undergo his transformation with my help."

Naturally, I was bubbling over with curiosity, and had more questions than I knew what to do with. I knew the psychiatrist had many questions too, but he pushed on, asking just one question at a time in a very calm, non-judgmental manner.

"Oh I see. Why Florida?"

At this point, Sophie looked up and made eye contact, clearly annoyed.

"Because I needed to rent him a boat. How else would he get here?" She asked, exasperated.

"Oh okay. I understand… Do you know how to get Florida?"

"No, but I have an address."

"What type of address?"

"It's my friend, Julie. I met her on the Internet too. She is going to help me."

"Oh, so you were going to go meet her at her house?"

"Yeah, I guess."

"Is she expecting you?"

Sophie just shrugged her shoulders.

"How were you planning on getting to Florida?" the psychiatrist asked.

"I don't know. Maybe by a taxi?"

The psychiatrist was asking for all these details, not because he truly wanted to know her travel plans, but because he was testing her thought process. Clearly there was some illogical thought pattern in this young girl.

"Okay. Well I wanted to ask you about something else, Sophie. You mentioned meeting your friend Red because he was undergoing some type of transformation. What exactly do you mean by this?"

"Nothing."

"Oh, so there is no transformation at all?"

"No…. there is. You just wouldn't get it." Sophie looked back up at us both now, evaluating whether or not she should trust us.

"Try me. I bet you would be surprised."

"No, I don't want to talk about it right now!" she declared angrily. It seemed that her mood had immediately and unpredictably escalated. Because she would be with us for at least several days, we didn't want to push it too early.

"Okay, no problem. But before we end for the day, I would like to play a short game with you, if that is okay."

"What kind of game?" She looked suspicious.

"I am going to give you thirty seconds, and I want you to name as many animals as you can during that time, okay? Emilee, will you write down her answers, please?"

I agreed and reached over for a pen and paper, eager to see how this would turn out.

Sophie gave a half smile and agreed to the plan.

"Okay, ready, on your mark, begin," he instructed and he started the stopwatch.

She immediately looked frazzled, but began energetically, "duck! Werewolf! um, um, rabbit. Um, um, um….dog!" She was stalling and stuttering in between animals.

She continued, "cheetah… owl… um, um, hmmm. Pheonix!"

After a few more animals, the doctor said, "okay, you can stop. Thank you. We'll walk you back to the rest of the group now, and will come get you later to talk to you some more."

She nodded her head and we all stood up to leave the conference room. As we walked back to the psychiatrist's office, he explained the test that he just administered. He explained that it was very informative that Sophie had had trouble with that test. He explained that she named far fewer animals than expected, and her choice of animals was interesting; many of them were fictional or "magical" and the order in which she named them was disjointed and clearly lacked a pattern.

When we got back to his office, he proposed that I try the test so that he could highlight some of these points. He timed me for thirty seconds and then analyzed my list. I had many more animals (my bragging point for the day), and he went on to explain that he could clearly see my thought process in the animals that I named.

"See here, you started out with 'cat' and from there it was logical to name many domesticated animals, as you did. Once you said 'rabbit' you moved to 'goat,' clearly signifying some type of transition. And then you named 'sheep,' 'horse,' 'pig.' I gathered you were naming farm animals—another related group of animals. The transition from domesticated animals to farm animals makes sense. Then after 'donkey' you said 'zebra,' as they are similar animals—another logical transition. Then you named several zoo animals after zebra. When I look at this list, I have a general idea of what your thought process was at the time. Now, let's look back at Sophie's. See the difference? She has no clear, predictable thought process, and therefore has trouble naming many animals at once. This is the definition of 'disordered thinking,' a hallmark of mental illnesses that lie on the schizophrenia spectrum. Does this make sense?"

I nodded. I was enthralled.[3] I couldn't believe a 14-year-old could be showing signs of schizophrenia. I thought it was a disease of late adolescence to early adulthood.

"Yeah, it makes sense. But she is only 14. Isn't that a little young for schizophrenia?"

"Yes, that is correct. It would be especially young, and very unfortunate if that were the case. But we will just have to continue to work with her and wait and see."

I nodded in agreement. I couldn't wait to go back and talk to her.

Later that day, we had a family meeting with the psychiatrist, the resident, a family social worker and Sophie's parents about her behavior at home the last couple of weeks. This wasn't Sophie's first time in the mental health system, but it was the first time she was admitted as an in-patient, and we wanted to see if anything in particular had changed at home.

Both her parents were seemingly smart and attentive. They were very concerned about Sophie's recent behavior, and not just her recent runaway attempt. She had become increasingly violent with her younger brother and sister, often hitting them for very small offenses, as well as becoming

---

[3] *Don't pretend like you're not planning this game for your friends at an upcoming party.*

exceptionally defiant with house rules. In the past, she would pace around the house when frustrated, or "when she needed to think," but recently she had been pacing much more often. Her mother said that in the middle of the night, she would often find Sophie pacing up and down the hallway, saying she couldn't sleep and needed to think. Finally, her parents noted that perhaps the most disturbing change in behavior was that she recently gave up her vegetarian lifestyle. Her mother said that she had always been a vegetarian, and was always very passionate about this aspect of her identity. For her to give this up was drastically uncharacteristic. Her parents reported that when they questioned Sophie about her new diet, her reply was 'that she was undergoing her transformation, and that it would not be convenient to be a vegetarian when the apocalypse came.' Her mother continued on and remarked that Sophie has always had delusions, and even imaginary friends that she would talk to (this is why Sophie had her own regular psychiatrist), but her mother's biggest concern is that she was beginning to act on these delusions—she gave up her vegetarian lifestyle, attempted to run away from home, and so on.

Sophie's story was becoming more and more colorful, but clinically, it was becoming less random and much more textbook. To the psychiatry team, it was becoming much more obvious what she was suffering from, and it wasn't good.

The following day, I was tasked with talking to Sophie a little bit more about this "transformation." The doctor also wanted me to find out more about the voices that she heard. Another hallmark of schizophrenia is audible hallucinations. The key to discerning normal imaginary play in a child and psychological pathology is the message that these voices give. If the patient hears nice, encouraging voices, this is more typical of a child's benign imagination. If the voices are threatening it is indicative of mental illness. The psychiatrist gave me a few pointers, including potential conversation starters and then wished me luck, reminding me where to sit in the room, in case things went awry. Yikes.

"Hi Sophie, how are you today?" I started.

"Fine," she replied looking away from me, and giving me the universal body language for "leave me alone."

"To remind you, my name is Emilee. I am the medical student working here for the month. How are you feeling?"

"Fine." Sophie did her absolute best to avoid eye contact with me. But instead of just looking at the table, she was shifting her eyes around the whole room.

"So what have you done in your group so far today?"

"Nothing."

"Really? Nothing at all?" I felt like a badgering parent on the way home from school with their disengaged 5th grader.

"Well, we ate breakfast and then we talked about goals."

"Oh, interesting...What were some of your goals?"

"I don't remember."

"You don't remember any of them? Tell me just one." I pressed on.

"I said, 'I don't remember!'" She yelled back. Whoa, this was going to be tough. She continued. "This is stupid. Can I go now?"

"In a few minutes. I just want to chat with you a little more. Is that okay?" She didn't give me permission to go on, but she also didn't threaten to leave, so I took that as my cue. "Yesterday, you mentioned a transformation you were preparing to make. I was wondering if I could hear more about this..." I waited for her to refuse. When she remained neutral, I continued on. "What type of transformation are you going to make?" The doctor had advised me to try and normalize the conversation as much as possible to encourage her to talk.

It was clear that this last question had at least piqued some interest because she made eye contact with me and answered immediately.

"Well, I am not like most people. I have special talents that most people don't have. And they don't understand them either. It has taken a long time, but I am about to make my final transformation into a—," she paused and looked up, "well, do you know what a werewolf is?"

"Yes, of course," I said, doing my best to seem natural.

"Well, some people change into werewolves, but I am about to undergo my transformation into a werecat." She looked up for emphasis.

"So you will look like a cat, and not a wolf?"

"Yeah, but not just any cat. I will have special powers. Well, really just the same ones that I have always had."

"And what powers are these?"

"Well it's too complicated. You wouldn't understand."

"You never know...Just tell me about one."

"Okay..." She agreed very hesitantly. "Technically I have three. Which one do you want to know about?"

I had no idea how I would ever actually choose one. I didn't even have the vocabulary to choose a magical power I wanted to hear about.

"I am interested in all three, but I want you to tell me the most important one to you."

"Hmm, I don't know what is most important to me. They are all necessary for my transformation. I will tell you the one that I wish I didn't have. It's called empathy."

I smiled inwardly. That's cute. I would like to think my empathy was magical too.

She continued on, "empathy is when I absorb other peoples' feelings and then feel that way myself."

I was still thinking this sounded rather endearing.

She further explained, "It used to be that if someone in my class was angry, I would feel that way too. Now, since I am undergoing my transformation, I feel what animals are feeling. When I see my cat at home, I feel her hunting instincts, and that's when I hit my little brother. My mom gets really mad, but she doesn't understand that it is because I have empathy, and I just absorbed what the cat was feeling. It wasn't my fault."

That was a curveball. I felt myself struggling for how to proceed. If I agree with her and "empathize," what does that make me? Am I supposed to endorse her delusions, or begin counseling? I didn't feel qualified to counsel or offer advice, so I decided to say the generic, "Oh wow. Well that must be really frustrating."

She nodded in agreement, and that was enough for her to continue on, "Well, you know. That's how I got Java."

"Oh who's Java?"

"I have had him for about a year. He is a raccoon. I rescued him from a fur factory farm. I could feel how scared he was and I knew he needed me."

Now I was confused. Was this a real pet? And what's more, does the fact that I am wondering if he is real make me delusional? I certainly didn't want to proceed by asking if he was real. Crap.

I decided to buy more time with, "Oh I see. What other pets do you have?"

"Well Java is not a pet. He gives me advice."

Okay, now I knew that we weren't talking about real pets, or at least I didn't think so.

"What type of things does he tell you?" I inquired.

"I don't know. He just tells me when people don't have good intentions, and that I should avoid them. You know, things like that." Naturally, I didn't know, but she continued on without needing my guidance. She listed off a bunch of different names and the roles that these characters had in her life. They all sounded like helpful, imaginary friends. I was starting to feel reassured about everything, but then remembered what the psychiatrist had told me to decipher.

"Sophie, are all of these voices nice to you?"

"Yeah, basically." She shrugged her shoulders. I then saw pure terror flash before her eyes, and she followed up with, "but there is Birdie." Over the last couple of minutes she had actually become quite chatty with me, but now she stopped and looked somber.

I might have been pushing my luck, but I pushed on, "What does Birdie say to you?"

"He flies above me and always tells me to gouge my eyes out with a pencil. I haven't seen him in a while, though. But I swear, as soon as I make my transformation, he is going to be sorry."

I was lost. I think I needed to wrap this conversation up because I felt myself flailing for things to say. I was having a hard time remaining natural about the conversation. I didn't know what might be offensive or patronizing. I needed help.

"Yeah that sounds really scary." I felt so stupid.

She looked up at me then and said, "Do you believe me?"

Uh oh. I was trapped! Maybe I shouldn't have been as accepting of the whole conversation. Now I had to choose a side! If I said "yes," I might be ushered over into my own psychiatric room for the night. If I said "no," surely I would break the trust we had just built. In an odd way, I felt honored that she would even ask me. It was clear she had a long psychological history, and has probably experienced lots of skeptical (rational) people.

I decided on "maybe."

She looked at me confused.

"I just have never heard about these things before, so I can't really say."

She seemed to buy this, at least temporarily. I was feeling pretty good and decided to push my luck, attempting to switch gears to gather more information.

"So what is your relationship like with your family?"

"This is stupid. Can I go now?" And she made an aggressive move towards the door. It was clear my luck was up, so I stood up with her.

"Yes, you may. Let me walk with you back to the group."

Sophie shuffled along next to me with her usual poor posture and didn't say another word, even when I said, "thanks for talking with me. Have a good afternoon. See you tomorrow."

She kept her head down as she joined the rest of the treatment group in their conference room. I smiled and waved at the other therapists and walked back to the psychiatrist's office. I was excited to tell him about the conversation.

We discussed the strong possibility that this little girl was showing schizoaffective qualities, which unfortunately is often considered more debilitating than the diagnosis of schizophrenia. Schizoaffective disorder is essentially schizophrenia combined with bipolar disorder. As her mother pointed out, she has recently needed far less sleep than normal (often pacing throughout the night), and she was also experiencing thoughts of grandeur (having the ability to transform into an animal). Both symptoms are characteristic of a manic episode, which is consistent with a diagnosis of bipolar disorder.

The bottom line was that this little girl was very ill. She stayed in the hospital for a couple more weeks, and eventually transferred to the outpatient program; however, the staff had little faith she would remain an outpatient. It was clear that she wouldn't be able to function in a normal school system in the fall and would likely need to go to a specialized academic institution.

I only scratched the surface of her interesting clinical presentation. We talked to her many more times throughout her time at Children's Hospital, and her thoughts and beliefs about the world became increasingly more scattered and delusional. Before entering my psychiatry rotation, I was largely naïve to the afflictions that face young children. As a society, we are quick to dismiss mental health problems and label the accompanying poor behavior as "poor choices" on the child's part. I can safely say this little girl did not consciously choose to be this way. In fact, I saw behavior in her that demonstrated her fight against it and some of her comportment was very consistent with any other adolescents. She possessed the desire to be accepted by her peers, just like we all do. She often acted out in her treatment group, yearning to be funny and interesting, reaching for peer endorsement.

She will face this struggle for the rest of her life. Mental illness like this is unpredictable. It could get better, it could stay the same, or it could get worse. It will take constant education, therapy, medication, and lifestyle adjustments to maintain it. Ultimately, mental illness like hers is just as debilitating as cancer, but it doesn't receive the same type of social support.

It is not easy to meet people like this transiently. I have no idea where this little girl is now, but I still think about her, and my thoughts are with her and her family, hoping that they have achieved some stability and happiness.

CHAPTER 9

The first two years of medical school are certainly difficult, but our sense of responsibility is largely self-imposed. We can perform less than ideally on exams, and as long as we are passing the course, we are the only ones who know the details of our grades. There are no patients to please and no physicians to impress, so our pride stays relatively intact. However, as soon as we step foot out of the classroom and onto the floor of the hospital wards, we stand much shorter. Much of our self-esteem problems stem from a little tradition called "oral presentations."

When I say "little tradition," I mean a custom that dates back hundreds of years. It is revered in medical culture, and its importance is so undisputed that we begin to learn how to do these oral presentations very early on in our training.

In theory, they seem easy, as the presentation is "just" a general summary of a patient and his or her problems. But take my word for it: these presentations are tough, demanding a very specific order and style. The ability to articulate and deliver exclusively medical terminology without hesitation is difficult enough, but the most arduous task is deciphering exactly what information should and should not be included in the presentation.

Playing Doctor

While the dreaded oral presentations are an integral part of all specialties of medicine, they are particularly relevant in internal medicine, and they are emphasized accordingly. A student's internal medicine rotation will typically be at a hospital and will consist of at least 12-hour shifts, six days per week. Medical students usually arrive at the hospital before their team's residents and attendings. This enables us to look up our patients on the computer, note any overnight events or lab results, and then go see them before the rest of the team. After checking in on them and performing a physical exam, we sit down to prepare our oral presentations.

In the beginning, I usually wrote out my presentations and read them verbatim, trying to avoid the embarrassment that an impromptu attempt might bring. Initially, this is an acceptable tactic, but over time you are expected to ditch the notes and report much of it from memory, using your cheat sheets only for lab values that would be cumbersome and unnecessary to memorize. These medical discussions occur while you are "rounding," or walking from room to room in a big intimidating group in which everyone is wearing white coats. Eventually it just becomes part of the daily grind, but I would be lying if I said it wasn't completely exhilarating the first couple of times I was a part of this group. Frankly, I had a hard time concealing my smile. By simply wearing a white coat, I gave off the illusion that I belonged to this group of physicians, but in reality I was just a huge nerd experiencing my first white-coat high, and internally I couldn't feel more ill-prepared and incompetent. And apart from feeling inadequate, overwhelming fatigue eventually dampened my enthusiasm for being a part of the rounding group.

Although it varies depending on who the attending doctor is that day, your presentation is often interrupted several times with statements like, "okay, move on, we don't need to know that part," or "whoa, whoa, whoa, you saw what on the physical exam?" There are also plenty of skeptical questions like "wait, what was their sodium? No, there is no way that is correct," and it is not uncommon to see a hand gesture clearly expressing that you need to speed things up.

Even if your presentation starts off relatively smoothly, these interruptions typically throw you off, and it takes all your strength to compose yourself in order to simply finish, as opposed to fleeing the group and running for cover. As a young student doctor, to work under this pressure and to perfect this style of speech while simultaneously reaching a reasonable conclusion about the patient's condition (complete with a practical course of action) is tough, and even writing about it now provokes some PTSD-like symptoms.

Often, these assessments and plans spring entirely from your own judgment; however, depending on your team's resident, they might offer to meet with you right before rounds to briefly discuss the patient and help you determine a plan. This helps ensure that your plan isn't completely ludicrous, and you can impress the attending doctor by appearing to know what you are talking about. Luckily, I had several of these helpful residents during my internal medicine rotation.

One morning, I met with one such resident just minutes before we were scheduled to meet the attending doctor to begin rounds. It was very rushed, and I had several patients to run by her. One of our shared patients was a diagnostic mystery to everyone at the hospital. He was undergoing a very extensive work-up (another term for "evaluation") for a Fever of Unknown Origin (FUO), and almost all subspecialties had been consulted and were involved in his care. Naturally, with his exotic presentation, I was very interested, and as an ambitious medical student, I felt motivated to crack the code. What a hero I would be!

During my discussion with the resident, she mentioned that we should consider infectious disease as a cause for his bizarre combination of symptoms. The patient was from a rural town in Colorado and owned livestock (including several llamas), so exotic parasites and other uncommon bacterial infections were important considerations. As an example, the resident mentioned an echinococcus (ih-kahy-nuh-kok-uhs) infection, which I later discovered is a type of parasitic tapeworm that can be transmitted from livestock to humans. It had been awhile since I had heard of this particular parasite, if indeed I had ever heard of it at all. (We learn so many things in the first two years of medical school that it is hard to distinguish between what we have forgotten and what we never knew. In any case, this particular infection didn't ring a bell.) At the time, I didn't ask for any details, but I should have, or at the very least I should have clarified the proper pronunciation. To me, "echinococcus" sounded a little like[4] "a kind of coccus" (see above pronunciation). Though it seemed a little bizarre for her to be so vague, I assumed I could think about this and figure it out before my presentation.

As we went about our morning rounds, we soon ended up at the bedside of the patient with the mystery ailment, who to my dismay was also surrounded by his family. Presentations are challenging enough, but they become even more difficult when they are done as "bedside rounding," an old tradition intended to make the patient (and often their family) feel more involved in the doctor's thought process. For the most part, I think this

---

[4] Actually, exactly like

practice is valuable, but as the presenter, you feel a need to censor the way you speak about the patient for obvious reasons. In theory, everything you need to say about a patient should be said in front of them because they should be fully informed of their condition. We shouldn't withhold information just because it is uncomfortable, and thus should feel free to propose conditions like "cancer" in front of patients if the situation warrants it, despite how daunting it may seem. Rounds and presentations are for brainstorming and collaborating, but naturally certain things are hard to bring up for the first time in front of the patients, so of course there are exceptions to the type of candid speculation that is in general encouraged, and some discretionary censorship always has its place.

Technically, my presentation that day didn't need censorship, but as it turns out, I could have used some censoring, as my lack of knowledge about echinococcus ended in smothering humiliation. To make my fall all the greater, I actually delivered my presentation relatively smoothly at first. As I neared the end, I started to outline my plan (really the resident's) to pursue a more extensive infectious disease work-up. "And based on the fact that he is meeting criteria for 'Fever of Unknown Origin,' and therefore infection is part of the primary differential diagnosis, I think we need to look into a....um....a....hmmmm (what did she say a again? Was it "a kind of coccus?" I meant to ponder what she meant by this. Crap, what did she mean? No she must have said something more specific. Was it gonococcus?)...a....umm...gonococcus infection," I mumbled almost incoherently. I quickly slurred over it, hoping they would intuitively know what I was talking about. Even if I had perfectly understood her, I didn't know much (or really anything) about an echinococcus infection, but a gonococcus infection is relatively common, and I just assumed that must have been what the resident had mentioned. I had thought it was strange that she would ambiguously propose "a kind of coccus" because that means close to nothing (and essentially just describes the shape of a wide range of bacteria), so given its ubiquity, maybe it actually was gonococcus? At the very least, "gonococcus" was truly a "kind of coccus," so I knew I wasn't wrong in that sense. I hastily went on to talk about a few more diagnostic possibilities and plans for further work-up, and then finished my presentation. I waited expectantly for questions from the team.

My attending nodded encouragingly at the end, but she said, "Okay good, but I just wanted to clarify one point you mentioned. What type of infection are you concerned about?"

Still not exactly sure what infection I was literally having trouble talking about, I quickly slurred over it once again, "I don't know, maybe, a gonococcus infection." I quickly went onto explain my thought process, "You know, just because he is around livestock a lot, and I guess, you never know - just to cover all of our bases." I thought I was just relaying the resident's thought process that we had discussed.

After hearing my response, such as it was, the attending doctor looked even more alarmed, "Wait, I am sorry… what are you saying? *Gonococcus?*"

I don't think she was trying to be overly critical, and still less do I think she was trying to embarrass me. She was just trying to tease out what I had said.

I shrugged my shoulders and sheepishly answered, "I don't know, maybe?" I quickly followed up with, "but I know, that is probably stupid and pretty unlikely." I truly didn't understand her skepticism. I thought maybe she was incredulous because this bacterium was so rare that she couldn't believe I would suggest it. It would not be the first time (nor the last time) that I would suggest something so implausible that it provoked this type of mystified response.

It was the first "kind of coccus" and the only "kind of coccus" I could think of. As it happens, gonococcus is the bacteria that causes gonorrhea, but I thought there must be more than just the type associated with the venereal disease. There is not. So, there I was, earnestly suggesting to my team of interns, residents, and attendings, *and to the patient and his family*, that I thought he had gotten gonorrhea… from having intercourse… with his livestock.

Granted, there are plenty of bizarre people in the world, and some have even more concerning habits. However, had this been a true suspicion of ours, this would have been one of those times that we would practice some censorship, and we certainly would have discussed this possibility before bringing it up to the patient.

The attending had the horribly strained expression of someone who is trying to mask a baffled smirk. (Looking back, I almost feel sorry for her. As entertained as I am by my ignorance, I am sure she felt twice as amused.) In a calm, and noticeably quieter voice, the attending continued to press my opinion. "So I am sorry. I am just trying to clarify what you think is going on. You think he might have a gonorrheal infection… from his livestock?" I think she was doing her best to genuinely decipher my thought process, but keep the discussion vague enough to protect the patient's pride.

When she finally used the term "gonorrheal," my mistake dawned on me and the reason for her confusion became very clear. At this point, I was profoundly embarrassed, to put it mildly. I looked desperately at my resident for help, believing she had gotten me into this mess, so she had better explain herself quickly. I needed out of this situation, and frantically panned the room for a lever to pull which would open a trap door in the floor. I have seen this work before in the movies (ok fine, cartoons), and was devastated that such an escape wasn't currently at my disposal.

The resident chuckled, fighting back more uproarious laugher. (It's generally not appropriate to be laughing hysterically at the bedside of a sick person with an undiagnosed ailment. In this situation, however, some laughter was warranted, or actually unavoidable.) "No, not gonococcus, *echino*coccus." All along she had assumed I had been trying to talk about the parasite infection she had proposed earlier. Apparently, I am a master of incoherence (this time on purpose).

Now the attending and the rest of the team were laughing. I finally had the nerve to glance at the patient. Unfortunately, now he was the one confused. I was still utterly humiliated. I couldn't believe that I had been confidently giving my presentation while my attending thought I was implying that our patient had intimate relations with his livestock. Luckily, the attending took over the conversation and explained the amusement to the patient and his family. Now they were laughing, and the patient swore his undying love for his wife, although he did admit to owning some very charming goats.

We all "enjoyed" a chuckle at the miscommunication, but my eye was glued on the door, wishing I could make a beeline out of the room.

Sandsmark

I felt like I had long overstayed my welcome, and besides, I had to go figure out what the hell echinococcus was.

Unfortunately, we never did diagnose his condition, as he was cleared and released shortly thereafter. As frustrating as this seems, it is relatively common not to reach a specific diagnosis in patients. And as long as their life is not in imminent danger, they are released with plans to follow up in the future.

CHAPTER 10

The crisp air signaled that fall had arrived, which also meant that I was halfway through third year. The red and gold leaves were radiant in the mountains; pumpkin spice lattes were in full swing, and Americans were content with the return of football. Well, at least some Americans. I was back in the Emergency Department working with my preceptor, and the ED isn't exactly known for its content Americans.

On this occasion, I was at the hospital for an evening shift and I distinctly remember trudging in at dusk. The sky was glowing with an orange sunset, and people around Denver were speculating that the sky's vivid color was a good omen for the Broncos game that night. I walked through the ED doors with a feeling of longing. I have never cared much about football, but my friends were all out together, and a beer and a chicken wing wouldn't have killed me. I knew I wasn't in for a night of football and merriment, so I was just hoping that the ED would be busy and interesting enough to preoccupy me for the night.

Whatever else may be the case about that night, it certainly turned out to be interesting. The start of the evening was fairly standard. I was able to see a couple of patients, do a few physical exams, present my findings to my preceptor, and at one point I stitched up a laceration with the help of an emergency resident. After a bit of a lull, my preceptor suggested I see a lady who was admitted to the ED, but was just waiting to be transferred to the hospital floor. My preceptor told me she seemed like someone who just needed some company, and since it was slow, there was no reason for me not to check in on the patient and talk with her a bit.

These types of patients, the ones that could "use a little company," tend to be particularly discontent in the emergency room setting. They just want to be heard, and while this is a reasonable enough desire, it requires time—one thing that ER doctors typically don't have. I am generally more than willing to step in and talk to patients in these situations because unlike ER doctors, time is all that I have to offer.

After stepping into her room, I started with my standard line: "Hi my name is Emilee. I am a third year medical student working with the ER physicians tonight. Do you mind if I talk to you for a while?"

"Well, I suppose I don't really have a choice now do I?" she responded.

Perfect, I thought. *I love when conversations start out like this.* "No, of course you do. If you are not up for talking to me, that is your choice, but I am in training so the supervising doctor sent me in to speak with you."

"Yeah, yeah, yeah... Fine. What do you wanna know?"

"Oh, um, ok…Well for starters, what brought you in tonight?" I felt like an idiot, and thought that my preceptor might have purposely put me up to this. If so, I understood why—conversations like this are important to experience and learn from—but it's an unpleasant experience nonetheless.

"Well no one can figure my shit out."

"Hmmm, how do you mean? What's wrong?" I asked.

"Everything. I have a constant headache that makes me blind. My stomach feels like someone has me tied up in a rope. I keep puking my guts out. My chest hurts, and my heart keeps skipping a beat." She paused, looking up at me, almost accusingly. "It's almost like I have done too much cocaine. Well at least back when I did it. You know?"

I didn't, but I nodded supportively and she continued.

"My back hurts so bad in the morning that I stay hunched over for the first half of the day, or I just don't get out of bed. Tylenol and Ibuprofen don't do shit. And my doctor doesn't give me anything to help because he doesn't care. I try to tell him, 'Ibuprofen don't do shit, and I need something stronger'… But nooo… I used to do drugs so I can't be trusted. Then on top of it all, I feel so dizzy that sometimes I have to lie down, and most days I am so tired that I sleep all day."

I wanted to focus on one thing at a time, but I didn't know where to begin.

One symptom seemed as good a place to start as any other, so I asked her to tell me a little more about her headache. As she continued with a convoluted explanation of her headache symptoms, complete with tangential outbursts about how the medical system had failed her, I realized understanding her medical story wasn't my goal. Like my preceptor had said, she just needed someone to talk to. So I let her talk. And talk and talk and talk, without worrying about deciphering the timing, context, and severity of her symptoms. Eventually we were back on the topic of her pain and her need for stronger pain meds, which led us to a discussion of some of her other problems. She was currently jobless, homeless, and drinking a lot. Just when I thought she started to open up and soften on me, she quickly switched tones.

"And you people are the reason I drink." She said with such disdain that I felt personally attacked.

I almost got up and walked out of the room, but I knew better than to take this personally. After all, I had just met her that night.

"How do you mean?" I tried to ask neutrally.

"Well, you guys won't give me any meds! So I have to drink!" Her tolerance for my "ignorant" questions was evaporating.

(For the record, emergency physicians will prescribe only a very short course of medication, regardless of the drug. A primary care physician manages any long-term medications and refills because of their regular follow up with the patient. In her particular case, it was clear why a primary care physician would not prescribe unlimited narcotics to her, but the ER docs were especially removed from her situation and medication requests.)

"And now, here I am without a hospital bed because they gave it to someone else," she continued. "Priority goes to people who don't do drugs, so here I am because I did cocaine once and was honest about it, and now I don't get a bed!"

I trust that I do not need to point out the absurdity of this accusation. My patience was wearing thin, but I was doing my best to keep calm and provide the best "I understand that this is difficult" face.

"Now I am just a frickin' science experiment..." she looked at me out of the corner of her eye as if I was such an eyesore, she couldn't possibly devote both of her eyes to look at me, "that they send little nursing students in to talk to!!" she exclaimed while flicking her hand in my direction as if to suggest "run along now."

Alright, that was my cue. I had absolutely no empathy left in me. I felt like I needed to leave immediately before I expressed just exactly how I felt about her. While I am sure no one could blame me on a personal level, this would violate my professional duties as a medical student.

I instead said, as nicely as I could manage, "well, it has been a pleasure talking with you. Feel better soon!" I promptly left the room, unwilling to hear any further rebuttal that she may have had.

I wearily walked back to where my preceptor was sitting. She looked up from a conversation she was having with one of the residents.

"So, how'd that go?"

I sighed heavily. That was all I had left. I was past the point of trying to fake a smile.

"That good, huh? Sorry…I didn't mean to throw you to the wolves. I thought maybe she could benefit from a friendly listener."

"Maybe. But I am not sure that would be me at this point." I couldn't shake the feeling that I had done less than my best, and that I was disappointing my preceptor in some way. She had faith that I could be befriend this patient, and I wasn't able to do that.

"Yeah, I get it. She is tough. This is certainly not her first time here. It sounds like she may be even more difficult than normal…"

"So why exactly is she waiting for a bed?" She obviously had plenty of complaints, but it wasn't clear what her precise medical condition was, and why that would warrant a hospital stay.

"Well, she was complaining of some chest pain, and had some mildly concerning EKG changes compared to her past EKGs on record. As you know, cocaine can often cause transient EKG changes, so it could be that, but given her age, her history of tobacco use, and her unclear medical history, we can't take any chances. Medicine [as in, the hospital's medicine department] wants to do a cardiac stress test, and observe her for a period."

I nodded, but I think she caught my frustration and skepticism because she continued.

"These patients are tough. Despite her having a pan positive review of systems, she does have some risk factors for true cardiac disease."

The phrase 'pan positive review of systems' is used to indicate that a patient is basically complaining in some form about every bodily system without any unifying symptoms. It becomes very tough to distinguish patients who are malingering and potentially looking for secondary gain (e.g., pain meds) from those that truly have an underlying medical condition. And of course these aren't mutually exclusive categories, and this is what can leave physicians burned. Consider the disgruntled woman I just saw. This was probably the 50th time she had been to the ER over the last 10 years, and so naturally her story becomes less credible and her "chest pain" seems unlikely. But the story is muddled with some EKG changes, which can indicate a cardiac condition. Since cardiac disease is so common, it can of course afflict even those who "cry wolf." You have to take everyone seriously, regardless of their history.

My preceptor and I continued to discuss her case a little further, and then we moved on to see a couple of other patients together. We returned to our computers about an hour later, just in time to see our favorite lady standing in the hallway looking sleepy and displeased. She had changed out of her hospital gown into her regular clothes and had her bags over her shoulder, seemingly prepared to leave. My preceptor peered over her computer and inquired, "Can we help you?"

"No, you can't. You haven't yet, so I wouldn't expect you to now."

My preceptor ignored her biting comment. I truly think these types of things don't even register with her anymore because she asked as calmly as can be, "Where are you going? We are waiting on a hospital bed for you."

"Yeah, well I am done waiting. This place is a joke. No one believes me that I need more pain meds, it took forever to get food, and just now I am in there peacefully trying to sleep, minding my own business, and these f*@king nurses keep maliciously lying blankets on me!!!"

While my frustration was genuine and strong earlier, there was no stopping my laughter at this point. I had to turn around from the patient and face the other direction in order to conceal it. (Subtle, I know.) I started to openly laugh, but pretended like I was coughing, excusing myself for water. If the patient noticed, she didn't let on to it. I made a mental note to talk with the presumptuous evil nurse who had the audacity to bring an additional blanket to her bed.

I was gone for a couple of minutes composing myself, and came back to my preceptor still grinning. I felt badly, but I really couldn't help it. I would have felt worse, but I knew my preceptor was amused too, despite the commonality of similar patients in the ED.

She laughed and smiled at me as I sat back down. "Well, she was a real treat, eh?"

I laughed, agreeing that she was a breath of fresh air, and then asked where she had gone.

"She left. We explained that it was against our medical advice for her to leave. I told her to come back if her symptoms persisted, and to follow up with her primary care physician. She agreed, although of course I think she just wanted to get out of here. But you know, we can't do anything else. Can't force someone to stay."

While the patient on this particular night was certainly an exaggerated version of the typical ornery patient, such people are by no means rare. No matter what specialty physicians enter, they will deal with difficult patients. As medical students, we are taught that, at least in theory, empathy should have no boundaries. We are to express empathy even to those who don't listen to us, appreciate us, or even treat us well. In fact, these are often the people who need help the most. This can be a tough pill to swallow.

Empathy is an interesting concept. It seems like a simple virtue that people almost cannot help but feel and act on, but it is a complex emotion, and it is not as natural or easy to practice as it initially appears. A lot of medical students, myself included, enter the profession in part because we feel we have a natural sense of empathy and we want to share it with others. However, we are exposed to such extreme suffering, and we confront it so quickly, that it dampens our ability to show empathy for other, less severely afflicted people. It is in a sense easy to feel empathy for the terminally ill and the acutely sick, and we see suffering of this kind every day. We see it so much, in fact, that when we are confronted with those who are less severely ill, it becomes harder to empathize with their suffering. Strangely, my empathy for milder illness was probably stronger before ever starting medical school.

I felt this progressive loss of empathy most strongly when I realized I could not even be unconditionally empathetic to my own *mother*. During my third year of school, she began having some chronic pain that was new to her and without an obvious cause. She had been exceptionally healthy her whole life, so this was devastating to her. Naturally, she turned to me for support, and oddly enough, I found it difficult to give. My first instinct was to tell her that in the grand scheme of pain and illness, this is nothing, essentially giving her the message "get over it." This isn't fair to hear from any family member, and it is especially unfair when that family member is training to be a doctor. It was as if my medical training was working against me: I was perhaps less supportive than a *stranger* would be to her.

I needed to hit the reset button. I was becoming the person that I told myself I would never become. I was reaching a level of burnout and cynicism that I always feared, and I was approaching it at a startling, unhealthy speed. I was only a third year medical student! My career hadn't even started, and for the next 40 years I will have to continually pull from reserves of empathy within me. I needed to develop a coping mechanism, a mental vacation that I could take when confronted with these empathy-draining situations. First and foremost, though, I felt like I needed to physically get out of dodge. I wanted a new surrounding, new doctors, and definitely new patients. And as unreasonable as this sounds for a third year medical student to want, let alone get, it was exactly what I got.

CHAPTER 11

I was in the "Rural Track" at school, which essentially means I was taught certain knowledge and skills, and was provided with mentorship and socialization experiences that together were aimed at illuminating the practice of medicine in rural settings and went beyond the standard medical school curriculum. Through this program, I signed up to do a three-month rural clinical immersion. This rotation would fulfill the one-month requirements for internal medicine, adult outpatient medicine, and rural medicine. (Every medical student has to do one month of rural medicine.) So I subletted my apartment in Denver and moved to Gunnison, CO for three months.

Even though I knew I needed a break (or more like a change of scenery because I would still be working), I was apprehensive about the change. I had to leave my life behind in Denver for three months. Set against a lifespan, this is a negligible amount of time, but I still wasn't thrilled about leaving my family, friends, and my apartment.

The organization that finds a host family for students hadn't found me a place to live yet. Usually, students in Gunnison live with the actual doctor they work with. She is a young woman who in previous years lived only with her husband in a big house, and so she gladly hosted students. However, this particular year she was adopting a baby. The baby was only a couple of months old, and so no outsiders were legally allowed to stay in the house for more than a week. So, I had a place to stay for a week, but I would be out of luck after that, so I was counting on the organization to find me housing in the meantime.

On the first evening, even though the doctor and her husband were perfectly nice, I felt incredibly awkward. This was nothing new or unusual for a third year medical student, but it is still very bizarre to meet the lady who will be teaching, evaluating, and grading you for the next three months as you simultaneously move in with her. For that first week, I felt like I couldn't relax because I was unsure if my behavior at home would somehow indirectly factor into my grade. Most nights that week, I returned home from the clinic and almost immediately went to my room, staying there for the night. My dinner usually consisted of dry snacks that I brought and stored up in my room. When I was feeling especially bold, I threw a frozen burrito in the microwave, but then quickly scurried back to my hiding place. I felt nervous to actually cook anything, lest I misuse one of her kitchen appliances.

Several days went by and there was no word about my housing. I was starting to feel anxious. I had no idea where they would put me if they failed to find a host family. I had heard horror stories, perhaps apocryphal, about students who had been placed in tiny cabins outside of Gunnison without electricity. I like to consider myself a reasonably flexible person, but I have to draw the line somewhere. If I was going to be working 60-80 hour weeks, with the need to study while I was not at work, I would at least like to be able to read by light instead of candle, and this is to say nothing of the weather, which was quickly cooling. Gunnison is the coldest place in Colorado, and spending my evenings chopping wood for a fire was too exhausting to even consider. I suppose this would have immersed me in true rural living, but I was more interested in learning rural medicine than rural survival skills.

As my first week was nearing its end, I received an email from the organization. They had found a place for me to live! The house was right in town, two blocks from the office that I was working in. How perfect! They gave me the address and told me to go over after work to see if it would be a good fit. I was so excited that I wouldn't have to stay in an outhouse that I thought little of the need to evaluate the housing assignment. I left work that day and, true to their word, I only had to drive a couple of blocks away. I got out of my car and was initially pleased. It looked like a well-kept, quaint little house. I knocked on the door and no one answered, so I walked around to the side of the house and looked over the fence into the backyard. There was a couple gardening. *How charming,* I thought, and then called out to them, introducing myself.

The woman looked up and gruffly said, "Oh yeah, hi. Come on back."

I let myself through the gate and stood behind them, trying to initiate a standard, introductory conversation, "How are you? Thanks for meeting with me… Beautiful day here…" No response.

Finally the woman stood up and said, "We will be right with you."

I thought that seemed a little cold, but politely nodded and smiled.

It is probably worth noting that these host families get paid to host medical students, so this is not charity work. If that were the case, I would have cut them some more slack.

After what seemed like ten minutes of standing in the backyard watching them pick vegetables, they finally stood up and showed me into the house. There wasn't much to see. It was certainly a small house. It was so small, in fact, that I didn't have an official bedroom in the house. (I was actually hoping for my own bathroom, but that obviously wasn't happening.) They showed me through the living room to a small den that was attached at one end. The den was separated from the living room by a pair of French doors. We walked into the den, my "room," where there was a futon—no closet, no dresser, no desk. To their credit, they did tell me they had a portable rod on wheels that I could use to hang my clothes.

They then asked, "So, do you have your own bedding with you?" Oddly enough, I did throw my duvet comforter and a couple of pillows in my car at the last minute, just in case.

I indicated this, and they nodded approvingly, remarking that it was good because they really didn't have much there. She then asked about a towel. Unfortunately, I had not brought my own towel, which is something I actually meant to bring but had forgotten. When I explained my oversight, the woman's annoyance was conspicuous. "Well, you will probably have to get one then."

I nodded my head.

"So how does this look? Would you need anything else?"

I didn't know where to begin. I looked at the grungy futon and then to the bare glass doors that left me exposed to the rest of the house, and felt like I was seconds away from bursting into tears.

The housing organization requires that host families have a desk for the students, and luckily I was able to quickly think of this. I would need to do a lot of studying.

"I am going to have a lot of studying to do. Do you have an extra desk or something?"

"Hmmm…" The lady looked perplexed at my request. "Well, we have our kitchen table you could use… I mean, you would have to move your stuff off it when you are done, but you are welcome to use it."

As inviting as that sounded, I wasn't thrilled by the idea of shuttling my things between my living room annex and the kitchen.

Then she exclaimed, "Oh I know!" And she turned to her husband, who at this point hadn't uttered a single word. "Hon, we could give her that extra TV dinner table that we have. Yeah! And that way, you could just keep it in your room. That would be much more comfortable and handy for you, I am sure."

A TV dinner table? Fortunately, I haven't eaten too many TV dinners in my life, but I knew the meals are pretty light and small. For this reason, TV dinner tables aren't really tables, but more like book-sized platforms, sometimes held up by four toothpick legs.

"Um, yeah, I suppose that could work." I knew my hesitation was evident at this point. I just needed to get out of there before I broke down in a more dramatic way. I know I can be high maintenance at times, and right then I couldn't decide if this was one of those times, or if this housing option was genuinely unreasonable.

I looked around for a moment more and then thanked them for showing me the place. I fibbed that I thought it would work, but that I had to make sure "that everything else fell into place," whatever that meant, and indicated that I would be in touch with them shortly. I left just a couple minutes after I arrived (not including my time watching them garden).

I was distraught as I drove back to the doctor's house. How was I going to succeed for the next three months if I had miserable (or at least highly uncomfortable) living conditions? What if I had to work nights and sleep during the day? They would be able to watch me sleep from the living room. I tried to reassure myself—I reminded myself that I was healthy and safe, and that is all that mattered. I could tolerate the room. I would throw myself into work, spending as little time at the house as possible, and when I wasn't at work, I would go to the library. I would study so much that my exams wouldn't stand a chance against me. Just when I thought I felt okay about it, tears stung my eyes. There was only one person to talk to at this point: my mom.

My mom is something of a free spirit who loves to camp, and she is content with minimal material things. I knew if there was anybody who could convince me that this place would be okay, it was she.

I called her, and when she answered I tried to say a few normal sounding things, but immediately started crying when she asked if I was okay. (There is no fooling her.) I told her all about the place, and said that I thought I was being selfish and high maintenance, and that I needed her to talk some sense into me.

"Absolutely not!" she exclaimed. "You cannot live there!"

I was a bit taken aback. I had almost convinced myself that I was in the wrong. My mom's reaction was both encouraging and discouraging. Encouraging because it meant that I wasn't being unreasonable and snooty, but discouraging because I still didn't have a house to live in.

She went on, "How could they expect you to live there?! Alright, who do I need to call to get this fixed…"

Of course, I appreciate that to this day my mom has my back and is willing to do my dirty work. However, I reminded her that I was almost thirty years old and that I would have my MD in about 15 months, details that pretty strongly indicate that I should be handling situations like this.

After hanging up the phone, I emailed the lady at the housing organization, explaining that I really didn't feel comfortable living in that house, and that I wanted to continue looking if possible. I offered to look around as well—I knew the quest for host families was difficult.

As I was considering my options, I remembered that I had an old acquaintance living in Gunnison. We hadn't seen each other in years, and we really didn't know each other well to begin with. Regardless, I made contact, and it turned out that she was still in town and amazingly had an extra bedroom, which she graciously offered. (As annoying as Facebook can be at times, it can also be a savior.) However, she had just gotten married and was going to have company on and off over the next several months, so it was not a long-term option. At least this bought me more time to find housing.

As if the hunt for housing wasn't frustrating enough, matters became even more complicated when I got sick. Really sick. At first, I thought it was just a garden-variety head cold, which is virtually inevitable working in a family medicine clinic for the first time. But then, while I was still staying at the doctor's house, her husband came home with a stomach illness, complete with all the bells and whistles. I didn't need a crystal ball to see my future.

I had already packed all of my stuff into my car and was planning to move to my friend's house that evening right after work. Throughout the morning, my head cold lingered, but at that point it was merely pesky. Later, walking out of the office for the day, I broke out in a cold sweat and waves of nausea undulated through me.

Confidence is sometimes hard to come by, but right then I was exceptionally confident—confident that I would soon be projectile vomiting. I hopped in my car and thought I would head quickly over to the new place I would be staying, but then thought the better of it after a second's reflection. I was only moments away from a re-enactment of my 21st

birthday, only this time without the tequila shots and expert dance moves. On what planet would an old acquaintance want to welcome a hurling houseguest to stay with her and her new husband? I decided I couldn't go there yet, and I really didn't want to go back to the doctor's house. Essentially, I wanted to do my puking in private. I desperately longed for my home. Of course, this was not an option, but I knew that almost as badly as I wanted to be home, I didn't want to be at someone else's house (particularly someone that I didn't know well).

Barely keeping the nausea at bay, I decided I had to splurge on a hotel room, knowing that I really couldn't afford it. I found a place in "downtown" Gunnison that seemed as likely as any to be devoid of comforter cigarette burns and long black hairs in the shower. I didn't even make it up to the room before I threw up in a trashcan downstairs. Luckily, it was outside and no one saw me. I was humiliated.

I can think of a lot of sexy reasons one may need an impromptu hotel room, but my reasons on this occasion were emphatically unsexy. I literally checked myself into a hotel room just so I could be sick there. I didn't know what else to do.

As I bowed at the porcelain altar that night, I wondered what the Gunnison gods had against me. My welcoming wasn't exactly warm, and I was convinced that I would never feel better or find a place to live.

Luckily, neither of those were accurate prophecies. In fact, the stomach bug (or gastroenteritis in doctor speak) only lasted about 24 hours, and I was able to move in with my friend the next day. The following week, the doctor offered to call her friend, who had a fully furnished apartment for rent and she thought it was available. It was in fact available, and it also happened to be the nicest place I have ever lived in. It was a beautiful, fully furnished, one-bedroom apartment, with a pellet burning stove, a full kitchen, a large living room (complete with Apple TV), and a beautiful bathroom. It was so awesome that I felt bad for ever feeling sorry for myself. I not only avoided spending my autumn in a living room closet, but also scored a gorgeous, private apartment.

CHAPTER 12

The stars were beginning to align and rural family medicine in Gunnison was becoming just as charming as I hoped it would be. For the entire three months that I was there, my job was consistent and straightforward: I would round on all of the hospitalized patients in the morning and then meet with the attending doctor who was assigned to hospital duty that week. I would present the patients and my plans to whoever was on duty, and then round again with the doctor. After this, which took about two to three hours, I would head over to clinic for the remainder of the day.

There are many pros and cons to both urban, academic medicine and rural medicine, and I'm still not entirely sure which I want to pursue, but one thing I can say with certainty is that I welcomed the change of pace in Gunnison, where the vibe was very relaxed. Often, out of habit, I would start my oral presentations with the same formality and speed (and anxiety) as I did in Denver. These were often met with a bemused look from the rural physicians, who seemed to be thinking something like, "What's with this girl? Chill out, would ya?" Soon enough, I did, and I loved it. In addition to the reduced stress load, my new schedule provided a great mix of inpatient and outpatient medicine every day, and there was also a great deal of patient continuity—

something that is lacking from shorter rotations in bigger cities. In fact, after just a couple of weeks in Gunnison, I had seen many patients (even outpatients) several times. It didn't take long before some patients would ask, "Where is Dr. Emilee?" if I wasn't around. It felt good, and it was exactly the refresher I was hoping for after feeling the onset of burnout back home.

An especially nice thing about working with one doctor for three months is that they begin to trust you. Instead of having a rotation that only lasts one month, with the first couple of weeks spent just figuring out logistics, and the last couple spent actually learning something, you get a solid 10-11 weeks of practicing medicine. I worked primarily with one doctor, but I also got to work with other physicians in the same family practice. Over time, they grew to trust me and even on occasion consulted me, asking for my opinion in case I had any ideas that they hadn't thought of yet. Of course, they were more than competent physicians (and ultimately knew far more than me), but I had just come from University Hospital, which is a large referral center that routinely sees very rare conditions. Since that was my most recent experience, my perspective on internal medicine was different. In fact, it was sometimes so different and "academic" that they lightheartedly made fun of me. When evaluating patients, I would often suggest incredibly rare diagnoses as possibilities for someone with a very common presentation, like an earache. They would look at me with a smirk that said, "Really? You think this young, healthy person with ear pain has an acoustic neuroma as opposed to, say, an ear infection?"

However, the truth was that we did have some patients suffering from mysterious ailments while I was there, and the doctors sincerely asked for my opinion. Maybe they were humoring me, but I was determined to have at least one outlandish diagnosis pay off and make me a local hero. (A girl can dream, right?)

One of these mystery patients was a middle-aged woman who had been suffering from seizures and memory loss over the last couple of months. Initially, the seizures were accompanied only by transient memory loss. In between the episodes, she would return to her normal self. However, over a period of just a couple of weeks, her short-term memory worsened drastically, and she began to experience personality changes. She had been a patient of the family medicine practice for years, and she had the whole group of physicians stumped. They had considered everything from malignancy to toxic poisoning, and seemingly everything in between. She had even been referred to Swedish Hospital in Denver (known for their neurologic expertise), but had returned back to Gunnison with no more answers than she had left with.

Now she was back in the hospital in Gunnison with an altered mental status. The periods of normalcy between her seizures and memory loss had become shorter and shorter, and during the week I was involved with her care, they had essentially ceased altogether. During this most recent stay, it was discovered that her sodium levels were very low. This alone can alter one's mental status and cause seizures, but it was still unclear what was responsible for her low sodium levels. Many medical conditions can cause this, but most of them had already been ruled out in her case. The doctors considered starting back at the beginning, repeating all of the diagnostic tests again, just in case one of the test results had been wrong or something had changed.

I became closely involved in her care. During the week when we re-collected lab results and repeated various imaging studies, I rounded on her every morning. I became fascinated by her presentation. Every morning that I saw her, it was as if I were meeting her for the first time. It was a real-life version of the movie *Fifty First Dates*. In the film, Adam Sandler's character falls in love with Drew Barrymore's, whose short-term memory has been affected by a head injury. Despite the obvious challenges, he still pursues her, explaining to her everyday who he is and how they know each other.

In the Gunnison scenario, I was a less-entertaining Adam Sandler, and it is safe to say the patient was not a romantic interest of mine, but every morning I would come in to greet her the same way: "Good morning, Mrs. K. My name is Emilee. I am the medical student who is helping with your care."

"Well, hi Emilee. Nice to meet you!" She was always very friendly and gracious, although not entirely lucid.

I would perform a daily physical exam as she waited patiently and politely, and then I would explain the plan for the day, at which I became quite good after several days of repetition.

"Mrs. K, Dr. (whoever was on duty) will be by in a little bit. We are still trying to determine why your body's sodium is low. So today, we are going to be very strict with the amount of water you are allowed to drink. You will only be allowed this one water bottle for the whole day. Any more than that could drop your already low sodium."

Equally adorable and perplexed as the day before, she would exclaim, "You don't say! And here I always thought that sodium was bad, and water was good!" This was usually followed by a little chuckle, and then she would add, "Hmmmm... Why is my sodium so low?" Interestingly, she delivered these lines almost verbatim every day.

As much as I wanted to say, "It beats the shit out of me, and unfortunately everyone else in the hospital,"

I would respond with a little more tact and sensitivity.

"I don't think we know yet, but we are running lots of different tests in order to figure it out." As challenging as it can be to form a meaningful relationship with a patient, and then re-establish it every single day, she was one of the most polite patients I had ever met. I had grown really fond of her, and desperately hoped my reassurances weren't empty.

"Oh okay. Hmmmm... interesting. This is so weird." This line varied slightly from day to day, but she always said something like this. By this point, I was usually at a loss for words, but tried to smile encouragingly each time, as if to minimize the abnormality of her presentation.

As that week's lab and imaging results returned with nothing abnormal, everyone was short on ideas and quickly losing hope. For whatever unwarranted reason, one of the doctors involved in the case had a strange confidence in me. Not long after the repeat results had arrived, we started discussing the patient.

"Where are you when we need you? You are freshly involved in academics and typically have lots of 'creative' ideas for a variety of conditions. Any ideas?"

I confessed that I did not. Despite my (questionable) aptitude for proposing the most outlandish of diagnoses for common conditions, here

I was faced with an uncommon condition, one with an even stranger clinical course and nothing at all came to mind. At this stage in her course, I had not read much about Mrs. K's condition because I had spent the last couple of days working on a small presentation for my attendings. (I did a number of mini presentations about various medical topics to serve as both a learning tool for myself and a refresher for the doctors in Gunnison.)

Flattered by the doctor's confidence in me, I decided that I would spend the evening following my presentation looking into various conditions that may fit the patient's presentation, but that we had not considered yet. Through the university, I had remote access to extremely extensive databases of medical literature, so I sat down that night to sift through some of it. I knew I would have to dig deep and call on the creative medical student within me.

After a couple hours of work, I stumbled upon some articles about autoimmune encephalitis, a condition that severely affects the neurologic system, and should be considered when other neurologic conditions have been ruled out. To me, it seemed like it was essentially the description of Mrs. K's medical case! When suffering from this condition, the individual's body mistakenly produces various antibodies that attack one's own central nervous system. Diagnosis of these conditions can be tricky because it is very rare, and even worse, there are numerous antibodies that can be responsible for the damage. Simply running a comprehensive panel of all the various antibodies will not identify an abnormal culprit. Plus, a screening panel like this does not exist. You have to suspect the presence of an antibody and then order just the one lab test at a time (which can be expensive, especially in the case of uncommon lab tests). For many other conditions, this is not the case. Consider the following example. If a patient presents with symptoms suspicious for liver disease, a physician can order a liver function test, and then look for an abnormality in the panel of values. In the case of autoimmune encephalitis, a physician must be aware of the exact antibody they want to test based on often subtle and overlapping clinical signs and symptoms. I wanted to present the possibility of autoimmune encephalitis to the doctors the following day, so I read up on several antibodies that are associated with the condition, and chose a couple that seemed to cause the symptoms closest to Mrs. K's.

I was excited to go to work the next day. I had butterflies in my stomach, and I couldn't wait to propose something that seemed both novel and fitting. I burst into the physician workroom brimming with anticipation. A couple of the physicians were already there for the day, so I enthusiastically began telling them about my discovery.

"So I was doing some reading last night, and I may have a few ideas for Mrs. K."

They turned to look at me, clearly interested, but probably more in the prospect of starting the day with some light comedic entertainment from the idealistic, impractical medical student than in actually discovering Mrs. K's condition.

I explained what I had learned about autoimmune encephalitis, with which they were generally familiar, and then detailed one of the antibodies that seemed most likely to be causing Mrs. K's problems.

I said there were only a few case studies, but these all suggested that the alpha-amino-3-hydroxy-5-methyl-4-isoxazolepropionic acid receptor[5] characteristically and predictively caused seizures, periods of intermittent confusion, personality changes, and sleep disturbances. I finished by noting that personality changes can cause people to drink too much water (a condition known as psychogenic polydipsia), and perhaps this was the reason that the patient's sodium was so low. We had actually already suspected this explanation because the nurses often found her sneaking water when she wasn't supposed to.

I looked around, trying to gauge their reaction. For the most part, they were nodding in interested agreement. One of them started, "Hmm, interesting,

---

[5] *What? You have never heard of this? Don't worry, me neither.*

and certainly a good thought. I am not even sure how they test for that particular antibody. We would probably have to send the sample away to the Mayo Clinic. That is usually what we do with tests that are uncommon, but potentially important. Do you think we should do that?"

I couldn't believe they were actually asking me to evaluate the feasibility of my suggestion. Essentially, the doctor was asking if my suspicion was strong enough to justify the expense. I wasn't prepared to answer this question. The excitement of my presentation waned, and all I could do was smile and shrug my shoulders. She chuckled and asked to read some of the articles that I had found.

Later that day, after she had read some of the same information I had, we decided to order the tests through the Mayo Clinic. My enthusiasm was restored. It would take several days for the test results to return, and the anticipation was agonizing. Of course, the conditions I had proposed were serious, and if they came back positive, it would be less-than-ideal news for the patient and her family, but I felt like some news was better than none, because as it stood, no one had any idea how to proceed. And, of course, I was excited by the thought that I might have cracked the code.

About a week later, I was in the clinic at midday when the physician who I had been working with on Mrs. K's case nonchalantly mentioned that the tests had come back, and that the results were negative (meaning she didn't have that condition). She went on to talk about another patient, but I tuned her out. I couldn't help but feel devastated. I actually thought that one of my outlandish diagnoses would finally pay off, but I had failed yet again, and what's more, a wonderful lady continued to suffer for reasons that escaped everyone. It was one of the low points of my rural rotation.

She remained in the hospital for a couple more days until her sodium levels stabilized. Evidently the austere water restrictions were effective, so she was discharged back home. However, everyone was confident that she would return shortly.

I actually never saw her again. Even after I returned to Denver, I continued to email the physicians to inquire about her condition, but the situation remained the same. She intermittently was hospitalized for seizures, confusion and hyponatremia, but no cause had been discovered.

I finally stopped emailing, but I can't help but think of her frequently. Up to this point in my training, I had strongly considered emergency medicine as a specialty due to the work I had done with my preceptor. I began to realize that this drive to follow up with patients, which was by no means limited to Mrs. K, would make emergency medicine very difficult for me because my curiosity about the fate of patients would never be sated. Initially, I never thought this aspect of clinical care was a priority of mine, but because its importance was becoming clear, my mind kept returning to obstetrics and gynecology. It had many of the exciting, high-acuity clinical scenarios that emergency medicine had, but it also had the continuity of care (on several different levels). I would have the opportunity to care for a woman throughout her entire pregnancy culminating in one of the best outcomes in all of medicine! In addition, I could care for women their entire life even long after their reproductive years as their gynecologist.

What was happening to me? I purposely requested to do my OB/GYN rotation first, so that I could *get it over with*, thinking I wanted nothing to do with the specialty, and there I was, almost halfway through third year, comparing everything else to it.

CHAPTER 13

I was disappointed that I was unable to solve the case for Mrs. K, but shortly thereafter I was given a new mystery to solve and I jumped at the opportunity to prove my diagnostic acumen (to use that word in the most liberal way possible).

She came through the emergency department of Gunnison Valley Hospital with a high fever and a cough. She was eventually admitted for fluid replenishment and further diagnostic evaluation.

According to our records, she had seen one of the physicians in our practice as an outpatient a month prior to this emergency visit. At that time, a doctor in Montrose (a neighboring time) had already diagnosed her with "atypical pneumonia." The term "atypical pneumonia" or "walking pneumonia" is used to describe pneumonia that is caused by bacteria that is not generally associated with a more "classic" pneumonia. The clinical findings connected to this illness can be different too. For example, this condition looks unlike typical pneumonia on a chest X-ray.

After the initial diagnosis in Montrose, she took a course of antibiotics and felt better for a couple of weeks, but the fevers and cough returned, so she came to us three weeks later.

Thinking that she still had atypical pneumonia, and given the fact that the patient did feel better temporarily, the doctor from our practice in Gunnison assumed that she just wasn't treated for the right bacteria, and sent her home with a different antibiotic, but with the same diagnosis.

Now, a month later, I was preparing to go see her and take her medical history. Before entering her room, I wanted to read the chart from the ED doctor involved in her admission. In her chart, the ED doctor commented that she was meeting criteria for "Fevers of Unknown Origin." You may recall this term from my humiliating gonococcal story. Despite my "experience" dealing with this problem, I still thought it was a colorful way of phrasing the problem, and one that would appear out of place when applied to other problems. Imagine if you brought your car to an auto shop with an oil leak, and the mechanic came back to say, "Okay, your car is all set. It seems that your oil is leaking from an unknown location. That will be $300, please." When a patient has a Fever of Unknown Origin (FUO), this means that he or she has had a fever of 100.9 on at least several occasions, that the intermittent fever has been present for at least three weeks, and that the cause is still unknown after being in the hospital for one week. This last criterion receives criticism because in many instances adequate outpatient evaluation can occur, so a person doesn't necessarily have to lay around in a hospital for a week just to make the diagnosis official.

With all of this in mind, an FUO is typically caused by malignancy, infection, or a connective tissue disease (like rheumatoid arthritis and other autoimmune disorders). I read in the ED doctor's note that he had dug a little deeper into her history, asking about recent travel, with the idea that certain areas of the country and world are more likely to have infections that we wouldn't see much of in Colorado. As it turned out, she had done some traveling in the southwest of the United States. Here, *Coccidioides posadasii*[6] is a relatively prevalent fungus and can cause lung infections. He ordered the appropriate lab work for this infection, along with many other labs, and he repeated a chest X-ray. The lab results came back as inconclusive, and the X-ray showed the pattern that her previous X-rays had shown, revealing nothing new or helpful.

Before entering her room, I quickly looked up FUO to jog my memory about the criteria and the various conditions to consider when a patient meets them. I was trying to consider the problem from as many angles as possible, but I wanted to focus on the rheumatologic (or connective tissue diseases that I

---

[6] *A medical student's dream diagnosis! Its pathologic features are specific enough that we are often extensively tested on it in school and on the boards, and it's rare enough to keep our interest, but at the same time, just prevalent enough that we may actually see it!*

mentioned) as a source of her fever. I felt so desperate to help this time around!

Between my first and second year of medical school, I spent a summer month on a rheumatology rotation. This was not required, but as students, we could apply for experiences like this and receive some scholarship money to participate. I saw it as a way to increase face time with both patients and physicians, which I did, and I also learned a great deal about rheumatology.

My knowledge of rheumatologic conditions had helped me some on the boards, but that was about it. Many of these conditions are rare, and I had only seen a few of them in person after my rotation. So, I thought this might be a good opportunity to dig into some of the more obscure knowledge I had accumulated in order to prove myself. There was a chance that I would think of a few additional tests or conditions to look further into. The drive to solve a puzzle that left others stumped served as a constant energy source for me.

My plan was to ask her a very detailed history regarding rheumatologic symptoms (joint pain, dry mouth, dry eyes, rash specifically on the cheeks or over her knuckles, etc.), and follow up with an equally detailed and specific exam.

I entered room number 11, where she was staying, and introduced myself. We started by summarizing her story up until that day. She explained that after the second dose of antibiotics, she again felt better for a week or two, but just last night, while grocery shopping, chills and rigors hit her all of a sudden. She told her husband that she felt terrible and had to leave immediately. She went on to explain that even with the temporary boost provided by the antibiotics, her cough never left her over the last couple of months. The fevers clearly came and went, but the cough persisted. It was mild, but nagging.

I began asking some of the questions I had planned in order to tease out whether or not this could be a rheumatologic, or connective tissue condition. She explained that she usually had some joint pain, but that it had modestly worsened over the last several months. She also reported that her joints especially hurt in cold weather, and that her fingers sometimes became whiter than the rest of her skin.

I perked up at this explanation. Sometimes when patients explain textbook-like symptoms, it is hard to conceal a smile. I know this seems insensitive, but it is hard to not feel excited when everything you study presents itself in real life. Or at least that is what I thought was happening. Immediately, a connective tissue disease called CREST syndrome came to mind. This is an acronym that stands for the various symptoms that it is associated with. I was especially interested in the "R" in the acronym, which stands for "Raynaud's phenomenon," which involves the constriction of one's blood vessels much more than expected during cold conditions, leaving the fingers white. Other general symptoms that can be a part of this condition are fevers, joint pain, and even pulmonary manifestations. This includes pulmonary hypertension. When severe enough, this condition can eventually lead to a cough. Her fevers, joint pain, and cough could just as easily not be related to CREST syndrome, but I felt like I had found a reasonable unifying disease process that explained all of her symptoms.

I hastily finished the interview (always a mistake) and went to prepare my note before speaking with the attending. With obvious excitement, I presented the patient to the attending, ending with my suspicion of CREST syndrome and my plan to order anti-centromere antibodies to test my theory. He was nodding along the entire time somewhat approvingly, and then said, "Yes, great thought, but have you looked at the labs that she already had done?"

"Yeah, I did. I just saw a CBC, a UA, and a pending blood culture, and then some of the infectious labs that came back negative."

"Oh, did you look at the outside labs? I think we ordered some rheumatologic labs back when she was in the office, and had to send them away."

Rats. I had forgotten about outside labs. In this hospital's particular computer system, there was one section for in-hospital labs, and then another section for labs that had to be collected, but then sent away for analysis. I didn't think they had done any labs when she came to the office a couple of weeks ago, and so didn't look closely enough in the chart.

Perhaps noticing my disappointment, he asked me to follow him and said, "Let's look. Maybe I am mistaken or maybe we weren't thorough enough at the time."

We walked over to the computer, pulled up the patient's chart, and navigated to the section with outside labs. I scanned them quickly, hoping that they had just ordered something common like an ESR and a CRP, which wouldn't be specific enough for CREST syndrome. Sure enough, though, they had ordered several rheumatologic antibodies, including an anti-centromere! Bummer. They had already thought of it, and again I was of no help. The results were all negative, except for the ESR, which can often be elevated with a number of different conditions, including general infection, so given that her working diagnosis was pneumonia, it was not particularly elucidating in this case.

"That was a good thought, though," he said, noting my change in energy. "You were clearly thinking about the right things. What else? Did you ask her any more details about her past medical history or medications?"

At the time, while I was talking to the patient, those questions seemed "lame" in comparison to what I thought was going on. The patient had merely said that "all that info should be in the computer," so I left it at that. I didn't want to solicit what I thought was unnecessary information *and* annoy the patient.

I explained to the attending that everything was in the computer, which I felt a little bad for because it was partially misleading. I hadn't personally asked her enough questions about her history because I had assumed it was all non-contributory. I knew I didn't have the expertise to pronounce this, but was too excited at the time.

"Okay, good. Well then we will just keep thinking about it and see what her blood culture comes back with."

With that, he walked away to the room of another patient who had requested his presence. I knew he wasn't disappointed in me, but I still felt like I let him down. I was also angry with myself for not being careful enough in my examination, and for letting excitement compromise thoroughness. My confidence sank all over again.

I pulled up the patient's chart and began to look over what the nurse had recorded for past medical history and medications. It said she had a history of childhood and adolescent seizures, and took phenytoin for prevention. It listed a couple of other more common conditions like hypertension (high blood pressure) and the medication for it. The chart made no mention of any surgical history, which was strange because when I examined her, I noticed a scar from a previous cesarean section. Such an operation should have definitely made it in the chart.

I had nothing to do until the physician was done with his hospital work, after which we would head to the clinic, so I decided to go back into the patient's room to get a few more questions answered. I felt badly about skimming over her history earlier, and now I had to basically admit to her that this is what I had done.

"Hi, Mrs. T. Sorry to bother you again, but I realized that I had a few more questions for you that I couldn't find in your electronic chart. Is it okay if I talk with you a bit more?"

"Oh of course, darling.'" She had a charming southern accent and was as nice as could be for her entire hospital stay.

"We talked about your c-section, but it wasn't noted in your chart..." She looked confused by the remark and was no doubt wondering how that could possibly be related at this point. I didn't think the operation was related to her current condition, but I wondered if there was anything else we had missed. "I just want to make sure we have all of the information we may need. Would you mind going through your history a little bit more with me?"

She shrugged her shoulders, which seemed to imply that I could continue.

"Let's start with your medications. Can we go through your medications together?"

As nice as she was, she looked at me wearily, as if to say, "This is annoying, and I can't imagine why this would be important." To be honest, I had absolutely no idea why it would be important either, but I was doing my due diligence, which I had technically reported as already done.

I had a print-out of her medications, and began reading them, telling her to stop me if there needed to be any changes.

"Claritin."

"Yep."

"Lisinopril."

"Yep."

"Simvastatin."

"Yep."

"Phenytoin."

"Yep—wait, no actually...I don't take that anymore. I take Keppra."

"Oh, really? Okay, we have here that you still take it..." I started to cross it off and write in the correction, and for some reason decided to be nosy. "Why did you stop taking the Phenytoin?"

"It was weird. It made my gums puffy."

At first, this sounded strange to me too, but then I remembered that one of the classic side effects of phenytoin was gum hypertrophy—the enlargement of one's gums. I hadn't met anyone who had actually experienced this side effect. I still wasn't thinking this had anything to do with her current condition, but now I was curious and pressed on. It would be a learning opportunity if nothing else.

"So, did your gums go back to normal after you stopped taking it?" I couldn't remember anything I had learned about this particular side effect.

"No! In fact, I had to have a dental procedure to have it fixed!"

Now my ears perked up and my pulse quickened.

Hoping for one answer in particular, and trying to play it cool, I asked,

"Oh really? And when was this dental procedure?"

"Oh, I think it was a few months ago, at the end of the summer," she replied casually, not understanding why I cared so much.

Bingo!

With obvious excitement, I tried to make sense of everything by summarizing what I had just learned out loud.

"So Mrs. T, just to make sure I am understanding the timeline here," I said, gathering my thoughts. "You were taking phenytoin for years, but ended up having problems with your gums, so you stopped taking the medication, but needed dental work in order to fix it. You had the procedure approximately three months ago, which would have been about a month or so before you came to the doctor for your cough and fevers. Is that correct?"

"Yeah, I suppose that sounds about right." She answered the question with some hesitation, clearly (and understandably) unable to match my excitement and sense of urgency.

"Okay, that makes sense. Well, thanks for answering those additional questions. Let me go talk to the doctor, and we will hopefully get you feeling better as quickly as possible." I was so anxious to go report what I had just discovered that I felt as if I couldn't get out of the room fast enough. However, as thrilled as I felt, I knew I had a track record of proposing unrealistic diagnoses, so I wasn't about to outline my thought process to the patient. I didn't want to imply that I had a diagnosis on hand when it might just turn out to be wild conjecture.

"Okay, darling, thanks…" She spoke slowly and in a way that implied she was thinking *what just happened here*?

I walked as quickly as I could down the hallway without actually running. I went straight to the computer station where the family physician sat working on his notes from the patients he just finished seeing.

I sat down next to him, and without even considering the possibility that he was working on something else and needed a minute, I blurted out, "I found out some other important history about Mrs. T."

He finished typing his thought and turned his attention to me. "Oh yeah?"

All the physicians in Gunnison were very informal, but he was definitely the most easy-going of all of them. I knew the interruption wouldn't bother him too much.

"So she has a history of childhood epilepsy, and was on phenytoin for years and years. In our system, it says she is still on it, but she actually switched to Keppra for seizure prevention several months ago because she developed gum hypertrophy from the phenytoin. Then," I said, pausing for dramatic emphasis, "she underwent a dental procedure to have the hypertrophy fixed at the end of the summer!"

"You don't say," he replied. I had his attention now, and he was excited—not as excited as me, but he immediately understood the implication of what I just told him. However, he must have sensed a learning opportunity because he asked me what I was thinking, as if he needed the full diagnostic picture.

"Well, I guess the classic textbook explanation for her current symptoms would be that she developed endocarditis as result of the procedure. The infection may now be seeding her lungs, and causing her recurrent fevers and cough. The various antibiotics have helped some, as most antibiotics would, even if they weren't ideal choices, but we aren't covering the right bug…"

Endocarditis is an infection of one or more of the heart valves and generally comes up in special circumstances; IV drug users, for example, are at very high risk for this infection, and those who have undergone recent dental procedures are too. There are specific bacteria that classically cause it, and since no one (for good reason) thought the patient had endocarditis, the antibiotics that were chosen for her "atypical pneumonia" were likely not the best options.

The infection is primarily on heart valves, but as blood passes through a compromised valve, the infection can be carried with the blood to various other sites in the body, which is known as "seeding." This process could explain her symptoms, and given her (now known) history, it fit the diagnosis perfectly. It was straight out of a medical textbook.

As I explained my thought process, he nodded approvingly. "Yeah, excellent. I agree. So what do you want our next steps to be?"

"Well the ED already ordered blood cultures, right?"

He nodded.

"So, then, we just wait for the results to come back from those, but I think we should also order a transesophogeal echo."

"Yep, fair enough, though I am trying to remember if we need more than one blood culture. I hardly ever see this. Something tells me we need serial cultures for diagnosis. I'm going to have to look that up."

He was lost in thought for a second, but then came back and continued,

"Nice work, though! I think you really may be onto something here. Did you notice a heart murmur of any type?"

I knew this was one of the classic diagnostic criteria, but I wasn't able to detect anything out of the ordinary when I listened to her heartbeat. I indicated this, albeit hesitantly. I have never been very confident about my ability to detect various murmurs, and I was hoping the absence of this physical finding wouldn't change his mind about my diagnostic ideas.

"That's okay. Who knows, she may not have one. We can listen together later." He typed a few orders into the computer, and then turned back to me. "Med student saves the day, huh?"

I beamed, not even trying to conceal it. I knew we didn't have the exact answer yet, but his comment was enough validation for now.

We entered the rest of the orders into the computer and gathered up our belongings to head over to the clinic for the day. I could barely concentrate because I was so excited and anxious to see the results of the echocardiogram and the blood cultures. Between every clinical patient, I logged into the hospital's system to see if any of the results were back yet.

By midafternoon we still hadn't learned anything, but the physician suggested we go back over to the hospital to check on the patient, and we could also stop in and talk to the radiologist about the echocardiogram images.

We ran into the radiologist right when we got there. He invited us into his office to take a look at the images with him.

He pulled up the images on his computer and explained to both of us that two out of the four cardiac valves looked free of infection. However, he stopped and zoomed in on the tricuspid valve, and then showed us the mitral valve. He turned to me and pointed with his cursor on the screen.

"See this here? There is some additional echogenic material here over both of these valves. Can you appreciate that?"

While I certainly "appreciated" it, knowing the implication of his explanation, I would be lying if I said it looked grossly abnormal to me.

"Yeah, I think I know what you mean…" I said, trailing off with concealed hesitation. He didn't seem to notice and continued, "Do you know if she has a history of rheumatic heart disease?"

"I am not sure…"

"Kind of hard to tell with the infectious vegetation that I am seeing here," he explained as he dragged his cursor of the point of interest, "but she may have some scarring on her valves, which would explain why she was at higher risk for endocarditis. But remind me, what are her symptoms? Why do you think she has endocarditis?"

I looked at the family physician to see if he might offer an explanation. I didn't want to be presumptuous and take over the conversation, but he motioned for me to explain the clinical history.

It normally makes me nervous to provide a succinct overview of a patient's history to another physician, but I was eager to explain this one. "Well, basically, she had a dental procedure at the end of the summer for gum hypertrophy secondary to long-term phenytoin use. Several weeks later she presented in Montrose with flu-like symptoms—high fevers, chills, arthralgias, cough, and was treated for atypical pneumonia because her dental history had not been revealed at the time. I think she was given azithromycin. She felt better for a couple weeks, then presented to the clinic here with similar complaints. Again, based on a chest x-ray and her symptoms, she was diagnosed with the same thing, but was started on tetracycline. Again, she felt better for a while, and then just last night, she was hit again with fevers and chills, and her cough has persisted almost the entire time."

The radiologist nodded, implying he understood the history and how it fit her current diagnosis. "That all makes sense. With that in mind, I think this is a pretty classic case of bacterial endocarditis."

"Yeah, and thanks to our smart medical student here, we figured it out," the family doctor explained and then winked at me.

Excited doesn't begin to capture how I left.

"Nice work," the radiologist said smiling, "we may let you stay here after all."

I laughed, thanked him, and then we set off to find the patient to explain to her what we had discovered. Endocarditis is not a diagnosis to take lightly, so we weren't exactly delivering good news, but almost any scenario is better than trying to treat an unknown ailment. The blood cultures would hopefully reveal the type of bacteria that we needed to target, and with the right antibiotics, she would be cured relatively soon.

When we entered the room, Mrs. T was watching "Let's Make a Deal" on what seemed like full volume, but she quickly grabbed the remote and muted it upon our arrival.

"Good afternoon, Mrs. T," the doctor began. "How are you feeling?"

"I feel a little better. The nurses gave me some more Tylenol an hour ago, so I don't feel as feverish."

He nodded and smiled. "Good to hear. Well, we think we may have some more answers for you now."

Mrs. T's eyes widened and she sat up straighter in bed.

"But first, do you remember our medical student, Emilee?"

"Yes, yes, of course I do." She glanced in my direction and smiled.

"Good. Before we go any further, I wanted to make sure you had met the smart medical student that has diagnosed you. We were stumped, and she figured it out."

Mrs. T made an "O" shape with her mouth and clapped with approval, and then grinned at me. I was elated.

"That's right. She asked important questions about your history that we had initially missed." He went on to explain that her dental procedure had put her at risk for this cardiac infection, but now that we knew what we were dealing with, we could more accurately treat her with antibiotics.

I was barely listening. This felt like the climax of medical school. Time after time, I had desperately wanted to contribute to a patient's care in a meaningful way, but up until this point, it felt as if every day consisted only of going through the motions of being a doctor. I simply imitated what a doctor did, all the while knowing that my actions didn't carry any real significance. I woke up early and went to bed late. I read about diseases, labs, tests, and treatments just to pass a written test or to make sure I was ready for the few times the doctors would quiz me. Patient after patient, I proposed one unrealistic diagnosis after another, dreaming of the moment when I stumbled upon something that they hadn't considered.

Receiving the praise from the physician was certainly rewarding, but it was the patient's response that truly touched me. She stayed in our care for a few more days receiving IV antibiotics, and then left the hospital feeling almost back to her normal self. She and her husband left a thank-you card for me (and a box of donuts), as well as their business card, urging me to stay in touch. Even if I had no other good day in medical school, it wouldn't have mattered. This episode, brief as it was compared to the duration of school, made all the early mornings, the long days, the dispiriting tests, and the crushing humiliations worth it.

CHAPTER 14

It was the dead of winter. I was back in Denver and I had just had three wonderful weeks off for the holiday season. It was one of the first extended periods since I had started medical school that was completely stress free. Last year's Christmas break, the one during second year, was tainted by the looming board exams, for which everyone felt pressure to prepare for over the holidays (even if they didn't), and this is how most breaks from medical school went: stress accompanied every nominal reprieve because there was always an upcoming exam to study for. But during the Christmas break of my third year, I was truly relaxed.

Thank goodness for that, because when I returned I faced the hardest rotation of medical school: surgery. This rotation is infamous for its absurdly long work hours, the regular 24-hour trauma call shifts, and the intimidating and serious surgeon supervisors. While I didn't have much control over my third year rotation schedule, I was able to request that certain rotations were at specific times of the year. I purposefully requested that my surgery rotation be during the winter. I knew I would never see sunlight, and I figured I would be less upset about this if there was naturally less sunlight to be enjoyed. Plus it was cold outside, so I would be indoors a lot anyway. I still think my reasoning was solid, but I had a couple of dark months ahead of me in any case, which would present me with a new set of challenges.

While there are many challenges in medical school, one of the most prevalent, and at times debilitating, problems we face is constant anxiety. Some people are naturally more anxious than others, but we all experience it to some degree a solid majority of the time. Our angst comes from a variety of sources; some of these are common to all students, such as exams and papers, but some are entirely unique to medical school—the third year clinical rotations, in particular, give rise to a special sort of dread.

Our rotations are anywhere from two weeks to two months long. After we complete one, we move on to the next hospital or clinic, where we have to familiarize ourselves with a new system and learn to work with new people all over again. It is like starting a new job every month for an entire year (and we all know how uncomfortable that feels). Usually by the end of our rotation, we are only starting to feel comfortable with the particulars of a facility. We've certainly learned some of the basic, practical components of the job by this point, like where we should park in the morning, where we should put our lunch, and what computers we are allowed to use. We'll also have learned the basics of the job, like how to use the electronic medical records for that site and how to work with the staff there.

And maybe, just maybe, we will have *started* to feel comfortable working in that medical specialty.

Of course, mastering a medical specialty takes years, hence the extensive residency training, but by the end of our rotation we do have a general sense of the questions we should be asking our patients and the exams we should be performing. We are aware of the very common conditions within that specialty, and we also know what ailments are especially dangerous, the problems that can't be missed. In OB/GYN, for instance, a urinary tract infection is very common, so we better know how to diagnose those, and an ectopic pregnancy is rare, but very dangerous, so we also better recognize this. As hard as it is to shuffle between the various medical specialties, we all understand that it is necessary. After all, it is the only way to reasonably introduce us to all areas of medicine in a manageable timeframe. So we continue to blunder through our clinical rotations, hoping we are sufficiently armed with medical terms and acronyms, but always dreading the next transition and the inevitable discomfort that accompanies it.

The change medical students experience when switching rotations is especially abrupt, but even single days can be characterized by an unsettling shuffle. For example, as part of my surgery rotation, I spent a week on plastic surgery. I was scheduled to be at The Children's Hospital and was there most of the time. One afternoon, however, the surgeon I was working with had the afternoon off. Wanting to ensure that I experienced plastic surgery to the fullest, she sent me over to University Hospital to work with a surgeon for the afternoon. (Heaven forbid that I might have the afternoon off too, although I could only use it as a chance to study.)

We wrapped our morning clinic up around 12:30 over at The Children's Hospital, and she sent me on my way to find a surgeon at University Hospital for a 1:00 surgery. I had to walk across campus to find an OR that I had never been to before. Once there, I also had to find the locker room and figure out how to get scrubs. Finally, I had to find a physician I had never met before and just hope that he was expecting me. (Forget that I hadn't eaten lunch yet, and would likely be tied up for the rest of the afternoon.)

Before I left I asked for general directions to the OR. The surgeon very nicely and graciously gave directions—instructions that no doubt seemed clear and reasonable in her head. "Okay, first go to the inpatient pavilion, and go in through the north entrance. Take your first hallway to the left, follow it halfway down, and take another right. You will see some double doors, and then proceed through the three pairs of double doors. Make sure you go through all three or you will get on the wrong elevators. Then, get on the elevators to your left, and go to the fourth floor. When you exit the elevators, go to your right...." At about this point, I was completely lost. I had stopped listening because I realized I couldn't remember which hallway I was supposed to take initially, and during the couple of seconds I took to try and remember, I missed a few more directions, so the rest of what she said was all but useless. (Naturally, the directions written above are more or less completely fabricated; I didn't know the directions at the time and I don't know them now.)

As she went on, I smiled and nodded, saying reassuring things like, "oh okay, yep, gotcha." Obviously, this only made things worse because she assumed I knew where to go. She presumably wanted me to succeed and find my way, and if I just acknowledged that I didn't immediately understand her suggested route through the labyrinth, I could have had her pause while I grabbed a pen and paper. But then again, that would show human weakness (which in this case would actually be human reasonableness), and I had to make sure I was ultra-competent in all domains of life. What if my evaluation at the end said, "yeah, she was good and all—always prepared for the surgical case, asked interesting questions, and had good bedside manner—but she had the audacity to write down directions as I gave them to her. Unacceptable." That seems like a rational fear for me to have, right? (At the time, this judgment seemed airtight, but in hindsight it resembles a pair of fishnet stockings—full of holes and definitely a mistake.)

I set off on my way with only a fraction of an idea of where I was going. I wasn't especially worried, though, as this certainly wasn't the first time I was headed towards an unknown destination on the sprawling medical campus. I also knew from previous experiences that I would be asking at least three more people for directions before arriving at my final destination, so I'd have plenty of company along the way.

Okay, I have thirty minutes. That is a lot of time. I can do this.

I entered through the north side of the inpatient pavilion. Check. One step of the directions accomplished. Okay, now what? Damn, I am already lost. I don't remember where I was supposed to go from here. I stopped at the front desk to ask if they knew the way to the particular OR and where I was supposed to go. Oddly enough, they had no idea who I was or what I needed to be doing (the nerve!). However, they gave me directions to a nursing station in order to ask. Great, more directions… I set off to the elevators and then after a short ride I exited to find some double doors. Oh good! There are the double doors that were mentioned in the original directions! There was something about three sets of them…Okay one set, two set. Wait, where is the third? (The nursing station was supposedly near my final destination, so that's why I thought I might have stumbled across the right area by chance. I just want it to be clear that I didn't mix up the directions I was told less than a minute ago. If I couldn't stay focused on some basic instructions conveyed mere seconds ago, the surgeon at Children's Hospital writing my evaluation probably should have reported my directional deficiencies as cause for concern.)

At this point, I was unsure how to proceed. Should I risk further confusion and continue to look for the locker room, or should I take some extra time to try to find the nurse's desk? Even though it was an added step for which I had made no provision, I decided on finding the nursing station. After some more wandering, I finally found what appeared to be the nurse's desk. (In any case, it was *a* nurse's desk; whether it was the one that I was directed to is another matter.) There they told me that I was one floor above the OR locker rooms, and that if I followed the main hallway to one end, I could take the stairwell down to the next floor.

Okay great, a one-step direction. I can handle that. I quickly walked down the hallway, hoping I was home free. On the way, I saw a classmate and was flooded with relief to see a familiar face. I wanted to stop this nonsensical quest and catch up with her, but I knew I had no time. I had 15 minutes left to find the locker room, get changed into scrubs, and find a physician I'd never met.

I got to the end of the hallway and saw said stairwell, but it required a badge. I wasn't sure why that was the case, but I saw elevators there too. I pushed the down button, but then realized I didn't want (and couldn't really afford) to wait. I turned around to take the stairs and held my badge up to the beeper. A reassuring "beep" sounded and I hurriedly hit the door open. *Shit.*

In hindsight, I never heard the comforting "click" of a door unlocking, which is theoretically what I should have been listening for. But in my defense, when you are not allowed through a door, typically your access is simply restricted, and you reassess the situation after you are denied entrance. Not this door. Instead of just not opening, this door set off an alarm. You know how alarm clocks are often forgiving at first, starting with a muted sound, and gradually working up to the wretched decibel that eventually wakes you up? Yeah, this was nothing like that. The alarm was like an air raid siren that immediately shrieked at my mistake. Hell, I knew I was confused and disoriented, but I was fairly certain I hadn't been drafted and deployed to a war zone…

I was on the labor and delivery floor, a section of the hospital that wasn't accounted for in the directions I was given to the main operating rooms. Giving the nurses the benefit of the doubt, I assume they saw the badges around my neck and thought I had access through all doors (like reasonable people would conclude, and like I had concluded when I held my badge up to the door). I of course didn't have access, and instead had just set off the "code pink" alarm.

There are lots of different "codes" in the hospital. I already explained the "code C," the one used for emergency C-sections, and there is the classic "code blue," which indicates cardiac arrest. There is also a "code red" for fires and a number of other codes that herald a variety of emergencies, medical or otherwise. The warning I had triggered, "code pink," is used for stolen babies, so as far as the alarm (and subsequently the entire hospital) was concerned, I had just kidnapped a baby and was on the run. As it happens, my initial instinct was to do just that—run (not kidnap a baby)—as fast I could. Like the stereotypical criminal caught *in flagrante delicto*, I looked to my left and lunged that way. I then looked back to my right, thought this might be the better way out, and then leapt in that direction instead. This flailing lasted a second or two, but then I stopped and realized that, not only had I turned into a cartoon character, but also that if I continued with my current escape plan, I was just going to make someone's job harder than it had to be. Security would get to the site, not see anyone, and actually think that a kidnapping was underway. I would just have to stand here, wait for security, and fess up. Bummer. It was only a matter of seconds before a nurse and security personnel crashed through two doors further down the hallway. I was impressed by their response time. I raised both hands in the air signaling, "It was me. I am ignorant and lost, but more importantly I am unarmed and have no baby in my arms."

When they saw that it was me, they smiled (thank God), let me through the doors, and then turned around to go disarm the alarms.

Okay, 12:48, twelve minutes to find the locker rooms, figure out how to get scrubs, and find the OR. *Ugh, I hate this!*

Unbelievably, I finally figured out the rest of the details, and went flying down to the OR. It was 1:05. I walked as fast as I could without running down to OR 15, the room in which the surgeon was working, at least according to the computerized surgical board. (I didn't have time to confirm this with anyone.) I peered through the windows of OR 15 and saw the surgical staff huddled around the operating table. It is especially hard to identify people in their blue surgical gowns, caps, and protective glasses, but I had never met this surgeon before, so I wouldn't be doing any recognizing anyway.

I was surprised that they already appeared to be working just five minutes past the supposed start time of the operation—usually it takes a while to prep the patient. The operating rooms are the surgeon's temple, and to enter the sacred territory uninvited is a very uncomfortable feeling, especially when you are late… Working or not, I had no choice; I had to enter the room and ask, so in I went.

No one even looked up. This was both good and bad—good that I hadn't immediately outraged someone at my mere presence, but bad because now I was going to have to get their attention.

"Excuse me? I am so sorry to interrupt…My name is Emilee and I am a third year medical student. (We are always supposed to introduce ourselves, but usually this is met with a look that says, "I don't give a rat's ass who you are." This isn't necessarily mean—they just truly don't care.) Is Dr. Heinz by chance in here?"

"Nope, not yet. His case is next."

Okay, good. That didn't tell me where he was or what I was supposed to be doing, but at least I wasn't late for his case. I went back to the main surgical control room. There were lots of people in there, and I began staring at their badges (trying to play it off as natural) to see if one said "Dr. Heinz." Luckily, it only took a couple of furtive glances to find him. Finally!

I introduced myself, and he was certainly nice enough and welcoming, but then said, "Oh, didn't anyone tell you? Our case got delayed. It doesn't start until three." I didn't know if I wanted to celebrate or scream in frustration. You mean I just experienced constant anxiety for the last 40 minutes for nothing? I could have taken my time, sauntered over here, and actually thought through my actions?

I didn't scream. I didn't cry. (I was attempting to pose as an adult.) I simply said, "Oh, no, I didn't realize that. Okay, great, thank you. Should I just meet you back up here at three then?"

"Yeah, that sounds great."

As with all frustrations, I had to convince myself that all's well that ends well. It's a challenge and a struggle and I don't always successfully convince myself, but ultimately you must push forward and assess your current situation without reference to the past. And in this particular case, I had more pressing matters to attend to. It was definitely lunchtime.

CHAPTER 15

There has been a big push over the last couple of years to minimize medical student mistreatment. Traditionally, a rigid hierarchy exists within medicine—medical students exist at the very bottom of the totem pole, with interns just above them, and as you work your way through residency, you gain ranking until you are at the top, as an attending. While these positions certainly still exist, and presumably always will, there is growing concern that this pyramid of authority drives those on the upper levels to intimidate people on lower levels. This intimidation can manifest itself in verbal, emotional, and sometimes even physical harassment, and occasionally public humiliation is used as a method of "teaching." Before every rotation, we are reminded of the system in place for reporting these various forms of mistreatment. There is an online system that can be used to anonymously report intimidating or otherwise unprofessional behavior, and the system is primarily designed so that students who have been treated poorly can identify the offending residents or attendings. It's not really used to punish someone for any particular violation, but to record and track behavior over time to see if it is a consistent problem.

Unfortunately, though, this system can only be used to report residents and attendings, and it cannot be used to file a complaint against any other medical personnel. *If* a nurse, lab tech, or medical assistant mistreats a medical student, there is no way to report it, and *when* a medical student is intimidated and threatened by a scrub technician, one is without recourse as well. No one will know what happened, and scrub techs carry on, crushing medical students one by one. It may seem unfair to single out a specific occupation, but I, along with most of my peers, have been mistreated or intimidated by scrub tech in particular. It is always dangerous to generalize about an entire profession, and I have since met kind and helpful techs, but it is also true that stereotypes are often born for a reason. Although the "cruel scrub tech" isn't a stereotype that has gained much currency outside of hospitals, I can assure you there are reasons that scrub techs have been the object of medical students' less-than-flattering generalizations. If you never plan to work in an OR, it won't take any great effort to steer clear of them, but for those entering the medical field, consider yourself warned.

Scrub techs gown the surgeons, handle all of the surgical tools, and monitor the OR and the sterile field—the area where the surgeons are operating on a patient—to ensure that no one "breaks sterility." To be sure, this *is* a critical job, and because the techs are more than aware of this, they carry out their job with terrifying earnestness. In fact, they are often a great deal more serious than the surgeons themselves. This isn't a problem for patients, and ultimately that's all that matters, but the unrelenting solemnity with which they regard themselves can cause problems for medical students.

Learning sterile protocol is definitely a necessary skill, and as students we undergo formal, although very minimal, training. It is at first very unnatural, and like any learned skill, it requires practice. On any given day, how medical students conduct themselves in the OR is almost without exception the opposite of what the scrub tech wants (even if the day prior they instructed us to behave in the manner that they are now criticizing). If we decide to introduce ourselves to them, they give us a dirty look, as if to say, "Oh you pretentious medical student. We don't care who you are." If we decide to skip that part and avoid eye contact, trying to remain invisible, they will march right up to us and say, "Excuse me, who are you?" After apologetically answering the question, they will typically respond with, "Yeah... we need to know everyone who is in our OR, okay?" as if our unannounced presence in the OR, *their* OR, has compromised its sanctity. If we offer our sterile gloves to the scrub tech to lay them out on the surgical table, they will be mad that we didn't take the initiative to lay them out ourselves. If, however, we attempt to do them a favor and lay our gloves on their table (in a sterile fashion, mind you), they will undoubtedly scold us for our bold presumption. I have had several difficult encounters with scrub techs, but a few in particular are especially memorable.

One morning, during my plastic surgery rotation, I was in the lobby of the hospital with one of the residents on my team. We grabbed a quick snack in between surgical cases, and were waiting for an elevator to return to the main operating rooms. From across the lobby I heard an accusatory cry: "Um, excuse me! Excuse me! Are you scrubbing in here?" I turned around to locate the interrogator, and to empathize with whomever was being questioned. I recognized the person doing the yelling from the OR and the break lounge—it was a scrub tech.

She appeared to be looking at me. I glanced down at my scrubs and surgical booties, and felt my head to make sure I was wearing the proper surgical cap. All pieces were correctly in place. Surely, she wasn't talking to me.

She noticed the look of confusion on my face, and repeated, "Yeah, you! Are you scrubbing in here?"

"Um, yes?" I replied, making it into a question, not because I wasn't sure of my scrubbing status, but because I was mystified as to why this was important enough to yell across the lobby.

"Well, you are wearing nail polish. I'm sure you know this is against hospital policy!" Her inflection implied a question, but her tone was pure admonishment.

I wanted to say, "I am sorry. I am having a hard time understanding you. I see your lips moving, but all I hear is 'I am scrub tech; hear my roar!'"

I was in fact wearing nail polish. It was not only the type that the surgeons told me I could wear, but also the kind outlined in my surgical *textbook* as permissible. (It has to be polish that either isn't chipped yet, or doesn't chip.) Furthermore, and more importantly, I couldn't wrap my mind around why she felt compelled to urgently call attention to this matter. As a trainee, I am certainly open to feedback and direction, but I wasn't working in her OR, and if the scrub tech had a problem where I was actually working, we could address it, and in a more appropriate setting.

I started to explain that it was the accepted type of nail polish, but I couldn't formulate the words properly and ended up stuttering in the process. She took advantage of my arrested justification and repeated the line about violating hospital policy. This time, I just said, "okay, thanks," with a thumbs up signal. This gesture, of course, could have been misconstrued as sarcastic. I didn't really mean it to be, but if it was interpreted this way, I haven't lost sleep over it. I was more worried that I had let the resident down. It is never pleasant to be reprimanded, especially when you haven't done anything wrong, but I wasn't worried about the scrub tech's evaluation of me. I was nervous because she had called attention to my policy "violation" in front of the resident who would evaluate me for my grade. As we entered the elevator, I glanced at the resident to see her reaction. She was smirking, and then said, "Emilee, you are going to hell— you know that, right?" and then laughed. Her smile melted my initial fear of her disappointment, but naturally my fear of scrub techs was as strong as ever.

This episode quickly faded from my memory, but it was just a matter of hours before a scrub tech was on my case again. This time, we were actually in the OR, which is theoretically a more suitable place to address an issue than the hospital lobby, but the scrub tech's intervention was still uncalled for. It was the end of a surgery case, and I was standing next to the patient as we undraped and cleaned her, readying her for the move to the post-operative room. Sometimes I easily recognize what my role should be and what tasks need to be completed, but other times it is less clear how I can be of assistance, so I stand at the operating table, waiting for instructions. If I wanted to be lazy, I could de-gown, de-glove and go stand in the corner of the room and watch everyone work, but instead I try to make myself available by remaining close. In this instance, as I was standing by, the scrub tech came up next to me to retrieve something off of the patient, and then said "yeah, you need to move."

Naturally, I was taken aback, but I calmly responded with, "Oh, I am sorry. I am just waiting here to see if there is something I can do to help." Given that I almost always stand by the patient at the end of a case, exactly as I was doing, I couldn't believe she was so put out by me.

Without missing a beat, the tech responded with "no," and simply pointed to the side of the room where I needed to be.

The physician assistant that was in the room gave me a knowing glance, one that said "oh my God" and "don't worry about it" at the same time. This time, I wasn't so subtle about my frustration. With a little extra oomph, I ripped off my gown and snapped off my gloves, in an obvious display of "I'm done here," and stepped to the side of the room. (Man, I really showed her!)

After plastic surgery, I moved onto my general surgery rotation, and the scrub techs didn't improve. The only difference was that I had become desensitized to their poor treatment of medical students. There was one scrub tech on the surgery rotation who came with a warning from a student who had previously worked with her. With rare exceptions, she lived up to her reputation. Despite my constant fear that she would reprimand me in front of the surgeons, thereby compromising my performance review for the rotation, she actually came around at the end of the rotation.

During one of my last operations, she overheard me mention that my surgery rotation was coming to a close.

Astonishingly, she expressed something resembling tenderness. "That's too bad, Emilee. We will miss you." She must have caught my baffled look, and she continued with, "We liked you here because you were good on your feet."

I am still not sure how to evaluate this last comment. To say I was "good on my feet" isn't really a compliment in this context, and in fact it essentially bears no connection to my performance during a surgery. A large portion of the time, I simply stood at the OR operating table. However, I think the scrub tech was so unaccustomed to giving praise that this was the only combination of words she could come up with to express approval. I wouldn't exactly classify my reaction as flattered, but I took what I could get and I didn't look back, though it was tempting to savor the moment. This was the first, and very likely the last, time I would receive a compliment from a scrub tech as a medical student.

Chapter 16

As I mentioned, a scrub tech's opinion has nothing to do with my final surgical block evaluation, so I couldn't take their aggression too seriously, and frankly, I didn't have the energy to care much what they thought. During this period, my enthusiasm for medicine was waning quickly. I was in the thick of my surgery rotation, doing everything I could to just arrive to the hospital on time. It was not uncommon for me to be running on five hours of sleep nightly. I often arrived at the hospital by no later than 5 AM and I didn't leave any earlier than 7PM, plus I had a 24-hour shift once per week. I basically didn't see my friends or family for the entire rotation, and even on the rare occasions when I did, I was horrible company. I was either too tired to talk, or my conversation revolved around surgical cases; boring as I was, nothing anyone else could say particularly interested me. At the time, I felt like everything outside my exhausting world was inconsequential in comparison, which was of course nonsense, but a tired mind cannot think of problems beyond its borders.

I was doing my best to maintain enthusiasm for the sake of the surgical team and my final grade. At this point, no specialty grabbed my attention like OB/GYN and I continued to compare everything else to it. While my path was becoming more and more straight, it was still essential I perform well in other rotations. Obstetrics and gynecology is considered a surgical sub-specialty, and thus my grades for my surgery rotation were particularly important for residency applications. So, I was caught in a strange situation: I knew I had to do well because of my target specialty, but, having decided on this specialty, I was less inclined to throw my energy into an area of medicine I knew I wouldn't ultimately pursue. To make matters worse, the weather was dreadful, and if I was lucky I saw sunlight on a weekly basis. I wasn't exactly primed for achievement.

About halfway through the surgery rotation, I switched onto a new surgical team. It was my first week with them, and I had three weeks left to go. Despite a daily struggle to stay motivated, I thought I was doing an adequate job masking my fatigue and growing apathy. Even when the practice of medicine no longer motivated me, grades still did, so I feigned enthusiasm and used academic achievement as my fuel. The intrinsic thrill of learning medicine will only carry you so far, and sometimes pragmatic considerations are the only way to get you over the finish line.

Shortly after I joined the new team, the residents in the group decided to organize a "team lunch" (which just meant that we would all meet in the cafeteria on a break between OR cases). At the time, our team consisted of a chief, a mid-level, and an intern resident (labels used to stratify residents on the medical training hierarchy). Unusually, our intern that week was a substitute. She was replacing the regular surgical intern, who was gone on vacation. She was actually an emergency medicine resident, and she didn't participate in any of our surgical cases, but she took care of the patients on the wards while the rest of the team was in the OR. Occasionally such replacement arrangements are made, even though they require residents to cross into a different specialty.

It was clear that this particular intern had no interest in general surgery. She was simply there to go through the motions and fulfill her surgical duties for the week. And if there is one thing that a surgical resident hates, it is someone on their team that doesn't share their same burning passion for surgery. Since it was clear that the replacement intern didn't, the other surgeons blatantly talked poorly about her performance during the week, but they didn't stop there; they also began to say disparaging things about emergency medicine physicians in general.

At our "bonding" team lunch, our mid-level resident's annoyance with the intern had reached an all-time high. The three of us sat there, beginning our lunches as we waited for the chief resident to join us.

The intern was always very pleasant to me, so we sat and made casual small talk, occasionally attempting to engage the mid-level. Our efforts were met with "yes" or "no" responses only, keeping the tension at our table palpable.

Eventually the conversation turned to emergency medicine, and the intern looked at me and asked, "Emilee, you are considering going into emergency, aren't you?" I had mentioned my moderate interest in the field earlier in the week, but was apprehensive about admitting this in front of the mid-level who had basically trashed the specialty all week.

I mumbled "yeah, possibly" in an attempt to placate both of them. The mid-level looked at me and spoke his first full sentence of the lunch: "you would be good at emergency."

I tried to smile politely, but the implication of his statement was all too clear, and I quickly looked down at my sandwich. My lunch went from delicious to nauseating in a second.

The intern stepped away for a moment to go grab some utensils. The silence at the table was so uncomfortable that I was obligated to break it, although I still don't know why I felt any responsibility to keep the conversation alive after the mid-level's remark.

"So what do you think makes a good ER doc?" I asked, hoping that there was some explanation of his statement that wasn't insulting. Maybe he actually held ER doctors in high esteem, and his offensive comments all week were simply a side effect of being fed up with the intern.

He looked at me squarely and said, "Well, you don't seem to care that you bother people with your questions."

He said it calmly and matter-of-factly, as if I had asked him for the time.

He went on, "And to be an ER doc, you don't really have to know anything about anything, you know? So it's kind of nice."

Whoa! What? In one fell swoop, he explained that I was not only annoying, but stupid—a medical student's worst nightmare.

Now my attention was solely on my sandwich and I willed it to stay there. I was nervous to look up at him in fear of what may come next. Was I also selfish, and perhaps a bit ugly too?

He decided to be talkative at exactly the wrong time, and went on to ask if I was considering any other specialty.

I didn't even know what to say, terrified that whatever specialty I landed on would elicit a cutting remark. Somehow, I managed to squeak out, "I don't know, maybe OB?"

"Oh yeah, I can see that. I can picture you being really aggressive."

He sure had a knack for slaying medial students' hopes. I interpreted his response to mean that I was not only annoying and stupid, but also disruptive.

All of the work I put into choosing thoughtful questions, all the time I spent studying and preparing for cases, and all the effort I applied to blending in so that my presence was only known when requested, blew up in my face all at once.

During the first two years of medical school, I was concerned about starting third year for several different reasons, but one thing that haunted me in particular was my propensity to cry. I have thin skin and can be sensitive to harsh criticism, but surprisingly, and to my delight, I had held it together for most of the year. Patients who had touched me with their suffering or their successes provoked the tears that I had shed. But now I had reached a breaking point, and the depressing turn in the conversation was more than I could handle. My face flushed, and tears spilled over without further warning.

The resident looked at me and said, "Oh no, Emilee. You know I am just kidding, right?"

Wow, hilarious, I thought. *I had the pleasure of eating not only with a surgeon in training, but also a comedian. How charming.*

I nodded my head quickly to acknowledge his "joke," trying to pretend that of course I knew he was kidding. Maybe my tears could be construed as approving hysteria?

Just when I thought I was on the verge of recognizing the situation for what it was—a couple of mean-spirited comments that just temporarily upset me—the intern returned to the table. She took one look at my face and exclaimed, "Oh my God! What did you do to her? What did you say?" Her dramatic expression of empathy pushed me over the edge. These tears would not be subsiding, and to make matters worse, the chief resident was quickly approaching the table with his lunch.

I ran. Immediately.

I find myself wanting to run from situations a lot, but in most cases I somehow convince myself that adults shouldn't bolt at the first sign of discomfort. This was not one of those cases. I ran as fast as I could, across the entire cafeteria into the comfort of the closest bathroom stall.

There, I quickly tried to compose myself, and realized two things about myself: I was as sensitive to criticism as I thought, and I was completely bonkers. I had just run crying from my general surgery team, the one team in my entire clinical training that would have the least sympathy for this display of vulnerability. General surgeons, and particularly the residents, have one of the most demanding jobs in all of medicine. They often work the longest hours, are proportionately paid less than many of the specialized surgeons, and are often targets of relentless harassment themselves.

I knew I was exhausted, I knew I was discouraged, and I knew that what he had said was blatantly wrong. But I also knew that I had to go back out there and somehow salvage my pride.

After a few more minutes of tears and deliberate deep breathing, I cautiously opened the stall door, looked both ways to make sure there wasn't anyone I knew in the bathroom, and walked over to the mirror to survey the damage of my emotional outburst.

Ugh. There was no denying that I had just cried my eyes out. I took some dampened paper towels and began to blot my face. Luckily, I am not up for applying make-up at 4:30 in the morning before heading to the hospital, so the clean-up wasn't as difficult as it could have been.

I stayed there for a couple more minutes taking deep breaths, and then prepared myself for re-entrance into the cafeteria. I cautiously walked back to the table, mentally repeating the mantra, "You're okay. You're okay. You're okay."

I was terrified to make eye contact with them. I kept my eyes directed towards my seat at the table, willing myself to take the remaining few steps.

But there, at my place, was a packaged, heart-shaped cookie with a note on top. My inner third grader automatically smiled at the sight of a treat. On the note, it said, "Emilee, I am so sorry," and was signed by the resident. I nervously laughed out loud. I was partially embarrassed by the gesture of goodwill. I had just been given a cookie to abate my sadness. On the other hand, I was relieved that he had found his words egregious enough to warrant an immediate apology.

I looked at the residents, smiled, and quickly said, "It's okay. Really. I am sorry. I think I am just tired," waving my hand as I spoke to further trivialize the situation.

The offending resident said, "No, really, I am sorry. I didn't mean it. I was in a bad mood, attempting to make a joke to ease the tension, and realized that this wasn't funny, and my poor mood has nothing to do with you anyways. I am really sorry."

And that was that. The chief resident went onto "pimp" me about the upcoming surgical case we had, which fortunately I had prepared for, so knew the answers to his questions. And the lunch nightmare was put to rest.

Arguably, this episode became a blessing in disguise. The resident who was notorious for being rough on medical students knew he had made a mistake, so he treated me kindly for the rest of my rotation. Granted, I would have preferred to elicit this treatment without creating a scene, but I had to take what I could get.

Did I have the ability to report him for being unprofessional? Yes. Did I have reason to report him? I think so. Did I report him? No.

I didn't because while I did feel hurt and disrespected and knew that his comments were ultimately insensitive, reporting him might have also been insensitive. In my current role as a student, I can't entirely understand the type of pressure he faces daily as a resident. I can't directly relate, nor can I accurately predict how I would behave if I were in a similar situation. In order to call someone unprofessional, I think one must have a good understanding of the actual profession, and I think my understanding is fairly limited.

So, this time, I decided to use it as a learning experience, one that I could apply in particular to patients. There will many times in the future when I will feel inclined to judge a patient or feel insulted by their behavior. In fact, it has already happened several times. I thought back to the lady earlier in the year from the emergency department, who was frustrated and left against medical advice. I hate to openly admit it, but that night I felt true disdain for her. I was immediately focused on her narcotic seeking behavior and her biting words. There is no doubt that she had mistreated me, but I had not done anything particularly helpful for her either. I could not relate to her life on any objective level, but instead of considering the reasons why she was behaving that way, I focused on her immediate actions and how they affected me. We all know that life's stressors have a way of affecting our behavior. Keeping this in perspective and making an effort to understand my patients' personal struggles will hopefully allow me to remain more accepting of otherwise objectionable behavior.

CHAPTER 17

Too often, our superiors ask us to complete tasks that we aren't particularly comfortable doing. Much of the discomfort stems from the fact that we aren't doctors yet, and thus don't feel qualified to perform certain tasks, and some of it is related to the unease that comes with performing any new job. I think it is safe to say, however, that a medical student's anxiety can be especially acute when we are contemplating exactly what duties we are competent to perform. We were explicitly told in lecture prior to starting third year that our student medical malpractice insurance only covers us doing things that are "within our scope of practice." Sitting in that lecture, I thought about how unthinkable and outrageous it would be if I ever attempted to do something outside my "scope of practice." But after reflecting on this phrase with a little more care, the notion became increasingly vague. During the lecture, one of us probably should have asked what exactly is meant by our "scope of practice," and how we were to go about making decisions on the basis of this principle. Technically, we are student doctors, and so does that mean we can do everything a doctor does, but a little less well? That logic doesn't seem especially sound (or moral). Are there certain tasks we are prohibited from doing, and are there exceptions to these restrictions, or do they hold in all cases except for some outlandish emergency scenario? But no one asked for clarification or examples. We all just accepted that we would use our judgment when asked to do various clinical tasks, and if a task was "outside our scope of practice," we would be sure to speak up.

In reality, our scope of practice is not so clear-cut. As soon as we are on the wards, away from our peers, we have no one to compare ourselves to anymore, and the range of practices we are allowed to perform becomes muddled.

Consider the following questions from various residents in different rotations:

Can you go change that post-operative bandage? *Yeah, that seems pretty reasonable. That surely is within my scope.*

Can you start an IV on that gentleman? *I don't know. Am I supposed to be able to do this? We did have one workshop during first year, where we practiced on each other. I suppose I could give it a shot for my second time...*

Can you go independently stitch that foot laceration? *I don't want to say no, or else no one will ever offer again. Do other medical students accept these tasks?*

It is complicated, and it is further complicated by the fact that we yearn to feel competent. We want to be helpful to both the residents and the patients, and we *need* to learn how to do these procedures. We want to carry out at least one task from start to finish, autonomously. And finally, we want a good grade for the rotation, which depends almost entirely on what the supervising doctors think about our work. So, we end up accepting jobs that are frightening and foreign to us.

For instance, during my general surgery rotation, a resident asked if I would go change a patient's wound vacuum.[7] A wound vacuum is a device used to close very large gaping wounds, as sutures are not always advisable or possible to use. In circumstances where infection is already suspected or a very likely complication, the last thing you want to do is stitch the infection closed and let the bacteria fester under the closed skin. Thus, the wound is left open, and it eventually heals via secondary intention, or from "the bottom up." A wound vac consists of a sponge, which is placed over the wound, attached to the skin by various adhesive layers, and then connected to a tube that is plugged into a machine that applies negative pressure, essentially sucking and squeezing the sides of a wound together. This ultimately promotes faster healing of gaping wounds. It sounds simple enough, but there are many steps involved in changing one of these devices. The individual steps are not necessarily complicated, but they take practice and repetition.

Before every clinical rotation, we are given learning objectives for the field we are about to enter. These objectives outline concepts we should have a solid

---

[7] *This is just as gross and scary as it sounds.*

understanding of, as well as experience we should have, in order to achieve competency in that area of medicine and do well on our final exam. My general surgery rotation was no different. One of my objectives indicated that by the end of my surgery rotation, I should "be comfortable with wound vac care and management." How we are to understand this and to what extent, however, is not exactly obvious.

In fact, learning objectives are often comically vague. I remember one that implored me to "appreciate the challenges that individuals face with access to care in a medically underserved community." Um, okay? Noted...and I guess, appreciated. I couldn't wait for the exam. I pictured a multiple-choice question that read something like this: How do you feel about the access-to-care challenges that are unique to individuals in rural communities? A) I don't care B) I wish I knew C) I greatly appreciate them D) None of the above. I had this exam in the bag...

With the "surgical wound vac" learning objective in mind, and the fact that I had already seen a couple of them changed, I assumed it was my time to change one independently—and perhaps it was. Still, after the resident asked if I would do this, I hesitated, searching his face for a sign that he was joking or would finish his request by saying he would help me.

Nope, he was pretty clearly suggesting that I should be able to do this.

I replied, "Okay, yeah, sure... You mean just like get all the supplies...and then just change it...or exchange it... like last time?" I was stalling for time, seeing if I missed anything and hoping he at least might offer to supervise.

"Yeah, exactly. You know what to do. I wouldn't ask if I didn't think you could handle it," he said.

Oh no, the infamous sneaky confidence booster. Now I had to do it, *and* I had to do a stellar job.

I set off to the seventh floor of the hospital where the patient was staying, and when I arrived the nurse was already in the room with him. I explained who I was, and that I was there to change his wound vac, doing my best to sound like this was the tenth time I'd done this that day. It's a common joke among my classmates that if a patient asks us how many times we have done something, we reply with, "oh, you don't even want to know how many times I have done this." Obviously, this is highly misleading, and we would never actually say it to a patient, but it illustrates the medical student's dilemma well. We need to be honest about our status as doctors in training, but we don't want to come across as unqualified or incapable of performing whatever it is we have been instructed to do. And the truth of the matter is that any task that we are asked to perform independently for the first time won't be anything major, or else we would not be asked to do it; any procedure that could have complications or can't be redone if we butcher it is always supervised.

The patient that I was asked to visit was on a ventilator machine, meaning he was still too sick to breathe entirely on his own. He could understand everything that we said to him, but he couldn't respond due to the tube in his mouth that went into his trachea. Most patients that I saw on ventilators were heavily sedated and were not aware of their surroundings; however, this particular patient was much less sedated than I was used to. Despite the fact that he actually appeared alert to his surroundings, I still assumed, quite illogically, that because of his ventilator he wasn't entirely lucid and would have a hard time noticing his fumbling caretaker's (that's me) actions. I was pretty much using a two-year-old's logic, assuming that if he couldn't speak to me, he wasn't lucid enough to hear me. This is how I used to lose games of hide-and-seek: I just covered my own eyes and presumed that because I couldn't see anything, I was invisible. So there I was, on the seventh floor of Denver Health Medical Center, trying to change my first wound vac like a real grown-up but still working via toddler logic. Stupid, yes, but this at least gave me a sense of comfort as I proceeded with my task, and, at the time, that felt more important than correctly applying commonsense.

I wasn't even entirely sure of the supplies that I would need to change the wound vac. I asked the nurse, "Can I please have a wound vac kit?" and just hoped that something like this existed.

She replied, "yeah, of course. I'll grab one." Oh thank God, I successfully completed step one and my pride was still intact. She followed up with, "what type of scalpel would you like?" Oh no, I celebrated too soon. I didn't know I would have a choice on this matter. Did it make a difference? When I observed other doctors creating a wound vac, doctors used a scalpel blade only to cut the sponge, so it probably wasn't too important to the process.

Since, according to my absurd reasoning, the patient couldn't really hear me, I felt comfortable admitting that I didn't really know what scalpel to use. "What do you think?" The nurse confirmed what I thought by saying that she didn't think it mattered too much, and that she would grab what she thought was appropriate.

Perfect, things were moving along nicely. When she returned, I stumbled through setting up my supplies, and then commenced with a 45-minute wound vac change that should take about 10 minutes at most. One must transform into an artist when changing such an apparatus. You are given an oval sponge, but obviously not all wounds are oval. You have to cut down the sponge until it matches the shape of the wound. Sometimes you have to use multiple pieces of sponge to accomplish this task. I struggled with the scalpel for a solid 20 minutes, cutting the sponge and then holding it back up to the wound to compare the shapes. I tried to carry out my task to perfection, even though such a routine procedure definitely doesn't require this degree of precision. The task was further complicated by the fact that I had to work around his colostomy bag, which necessitated a little more coordination. A colostomy is a procedure in which a surgeon cuts the intestines and brings the end of this "tubing" (i.e., the intestines) up through the abdominal wall. A hole is made on the surface of the skin and a bag is attached to it. There are various medical indications for this procedure, but the aim is to allow a patient to have a bowel movement into a bag that rests on their abdomen. The sack is fairly secure, but nonetheless a bag of poop resting in your workspace is a little unsettling, even in the best of circumstances. Finally, with multiple sponges all laid across the wound, I taped them down in the manner I thought was appropriate. I stood up straight and stepped back to admire my work.

It looked terrible, like a pre-school art project only a mother can love. But as long it worked, the aesthetics didn't matter. I hooked up the tubing to the machine, praying the sponges would actually all depress and conform to the wound when I applied the suction. Lo and behold, the machine started sucking, which meant I had set everything up right, and the sponges all conformed to the wound, looking like one seamless, perfectly applied wound vac!

I smiled at the patient as casually as possible, but I was beaming on the inside, delighted and relieved I didn't have to admit my incompetence to the surgical team. Job well done for the day, and the patient was none the wiser. Perfect!

The resident on the team and I returned to change the wound vac together a couple of days later. The whole process is much easier with two people, and we were busy that day, so we wanted to complete the task as efficiently as possible.

The patient had significantly improved and did not need to be on the ventilator anymore, so he was able to converse with us as we changed it. The resident was having me do the majority of the work, which surprisingly (but happily) seemed much easier today; I wasn't the only who noticed my newfound dexterity, though.

"Well, you are getting the hang of this," the patient said. "I wasn't sure how it would all work out the other day when you were in here."

Rats. I knew that the "if he can't speak, he can't hear" idea was absurd, but I didn't think he would call me out!

He went on to explain that after a prior surgery, he learned how to change his own wound vacs at home, and acknowledged that they are tough initially. While he was nice about it, I was still a little embarrassed. The patient not only noticed my inadequacies, but also happened to be a pro himself!

Oh well, keeping with the theme of third year, all's well that ends well, but I still wished my first attempt at a wound vac change could have been on someone heavily sedated and not an observant expert...

CHAPTER 18

The weeks following the fateful wound vac gave me plenty of opportunity to redeem myself, and as I neared the end of my surgery rotation, I could whip up a wound vac with confidence (well, without horror and humiliation). I only had two weeks left of my general surgery rotation, but that meant my final exam for the rotation was also a mere two weeks away and unfortunately, but unsurprisingly, I couldn't feel less prepared. Every time I am able to overcome (or blunder helplessly through) one challenge, like the wound vac change, another one awaits me, and my anxiety is re-ignited all over again. This particular challenge, considered in isolation, wasn't such a big deal, but these things happened to my peers and me all of the time. A general sense of unease permeated almost every day of every rotation; it was no wonder that my anxiety began to manifest itself in my dreams. Take the following dream, which for some reason was set in the family medicine clinic in Gunnison, even though I had left there a couple of months before.

I dreamt that it was the end of the workday and I was one of the only people left in the family medicine outpatient clinic. I was back in the physician workroom writing patient notes from the day when one of the medical assistants (MA) came back looking for a physician to write and sign a prescription. They asked me if I could do it. Medical students are never allowed to sign prescriptions, but we are allowed to write them (if we are familiar with the drug and its directions). I explained this to the MA, who said that was okay, and that it would still be really helpful if I could just physically write out the prescription.

"Sure, what is the prescription for?" I asked.

She replied, "I don't know. I think it's for this malpractice type of thing. I don't really understand, but they need this prescription."

This clearly doesn't make sense outside of dreamland, but even within it I wasn't sure that I understood.

"Okay, well what are the directions for the medication?"

"Its supposed to be: Take one pill by mouth in the face of emergent legal action."

Oh okay, gotcha. That makes more sense. And in my dream it did, as most outlandish things do.

I started to write out the prescription, but kept messing it up, paper after paper. My handwriting would be illegible, or I would misspell words or leave them out altogether. Finally I had one sheet of paper left.

Okay, I thought in my dream. *Just concentrate on this one, extremely simple task. I can do this... Oh, but first I better put some lotion on my hands. They sure are dry.*

As you might expect at this point, I put too much lotion on my hands, and when I went to write out the prescription on the last piece of paper I had, it disintegrated before my eyes.

Great. Now what do I do? Hmmm...

Oh! I know! There is a cake in the backroom. (This part is believable. There are always treats galore in clinics, brought in by employees and patients alike). *I will just carve out the prescription into the cake! Duh!*

I set out to the backroom to begin my prescription carving. I sat writing with a knife, and as I neared the end, I took a step back to look at the whole picture and admire my work.

What the hell? This is an absolute mess! This is never going to work. Why didn't I just keep the cake intact, and write on it with frosting? Man I am just not thinking clearly!

So I took the rubble of the cake and tried to smash it back together into one whole cake. I then took some frosting and tried to write on the salvaged cake. This might surprise you, but that didn't work either. It was still completely illegible.

Okay, I need a break from this. It will come to me. Meanwhile, I had received a text from the attending doctor asking if I wanted to come over and watch a movie at her house (a totally normal and professional question, especially coming from someone I had just recently met and had only seen at work). I set off over to her house, and when I arrived I set my purse on a little workbench in the entryway. Next to my purse there was a bottle of Elmer's Glue.

Eureka! I know, I will take the glue and write the prescription onto the side of my purse. Finally, a solution to the crisis! As I was writing beautiful, legible words, the doctor's dog ran up to greet me and knocked the purse over, smearing all of the glue. The doctor was close behind to welcome me. She found me in her entryway, bottle of glue in my hand, purse on the ground, and crying...inconsolably. And then I woke up.

I was relieved I had been dreaming, but I still felt a bit uneasy. Even in the middle of night, the meaning of the dream, or what I took as the meaning, struck me immediately. It wasn't a particularly hard dream to interpret, and the symbolism was fairly obvious. Basic tasks can be surprisingly difficult, and sometimes you can approach problems in ways that are (or at least seem) completely absurd, especially when you are trying to find your way in a new and difficult field. Often my days are problem-solving nightmares just like the one recounted above. The only difference is that there isn't much cake carving on the wards.

CHAPTER 19

As a medical student on general surgery, it is an expectation that we complete one 24-hour shift per week. These shifts are usually on the weekends, and we work with the trauma surgeons who take any emergent cases that cannot wait for daytime OR scheduling. Despite their horrible and exhausting length, I usually enjoyed them. The cases that came in were always interesting and exciting (from a learner's perspective, not so much the patient's). Also, by this time in the rotation, I felt like I finally had a handle on what was expected of me. I was meshing well with the residents and knew how I could be of help to the team and the patients.

The night had been relatively slow so far, with no operations, but around 8 PM a victim of an abdominal stabbing came into the emergency room. After evaluating the patient with the resident, we deemed him stable, with the plan to do serial abdominal exams and blood work every two hours. The purpose of this was to evaluate whether or not he was bleeding into his abdomen. At first, he didn't appear to be, but the only way to check this without taking him immediately to the OR is serial blood work (to track his blood count) and abdominal exams (to see if his abdomen was becoming more distended, tense, or painful, which would signify an active bleed into the abdomen—a clear indication for an emergent operation). I was tasked with doing several of these exams, so I had faithfully gone down to the ER every two hours, for many hours. When I returned to the resident lounge after yet another exam, the surgery resident told me that he was going to lie down for a couple hours and that I should do the same. After all, based on his exams and his labs, the patient was not changing and seemed stable. He told me he would call me if he received any news from the emergency department to suggest otherwise. I was relieved by the opportunity to lie down for a bit. I went to one of the on-call rooms and set my alarm. It was 2:45 AM. I set my alarm for 4:50. I could be upstairs by 5:00 in order to start collecting information from the admitted patients on our service for the incoming day team. My job was to look up our patients on the computer and get all of their overnight vitals, labs, and any other recent events from the nurses to help the day team before morning rounds. I assumed that I didn't need to worry about the patient in the ER because the resident would call me if something changed or needed to be done. I fell asleep almost immediately.

After what seemed like 30 seconds, my alarm jingled. At first, it was incorporated into my dream. I was dreaming that I was desperately trying to cross the road but couldn't because there was a steady stream of bikers. Their pedal strokes seemed to perfectly match the tune of my alarm... I was finally shaken out of my comatose sleep to find myself in the dark call room on the familiar little hard cot that the hospital disguises as a bed using stiff sheets and thin blankets, neither of which I was underneath. As a medical student, I always felt self-conscious about sleeping in these resident on-call rooms. I constantly wanted to retain the ability to spring to life in case I was accidentally sleeping in someone else's bed. So if I ever did lie down, I always kept my shoes on, and usually covered up with just my jacket. That way, if someone did walk in, I could pretend that I had tripped and accidentally fallen asleep, instead of giving the impression that I had deliberately taken off my shoes and climbed under the sheets.

Turning off my alarm, I peeled myself off the bed and plodded to the shared resident bathroom to throw some water on my face. I looked at my phone again to see if I had missed any call or text accidentally, nervous that I might have with the way that I had slept. *I guess nothing happened with that guy from the ED,* I thought, noting no missed calls or messages. I gathered my stuff to go upstairs and begin my early morning duties for the team that would soon be returning for the day.

After gathering all of the info I needed and meeting with the surgical intern to touch base, we headed down to the resident rounds that were held at 6AM in one of the conference rooms—the location where all of the surgical teams met every morning, and where the night team would discuss any overnight events with the day residents. This is an arena where 3rd year students are permitted to listen, but not really invited to speak. Before we started, one of the chiefs noticed that Brian, the resident that I had been working with overnight, wasn't present and asked where he was. Someone said that they thought he was in the OR with one of the overnight patients who had just been designated to their service, and that we would discuss this particular patient in a few minutes. I thought I was aware of all the patients Brian was involved with, so this seemed strange, but I brushed it off, knowing fully well I was no expert on the logistics of how these various surgical teams worked. As a group we began discussing all the patients on the list. When we got to the patient that I had taken care of in the ED overnight, I assumed one of the other residents would explain that he was stable and nothing further needed to be done on our end surgically, and that he was just here now for medical observation. Instead, he began to explain the case, the beginning of which was familiar, but then ended with the fact that he was eventually taken back to the OR with an abdomen full of blood, and that Brian was currently in the OR operating on him with the attending.

My heart sunk. *What?! He told me he would wake me up… What happened? He must really hate me! I must have really messed up if I wasn't even invited to the OR*

*after I had spent all night with this patient. What the heck
was the point of this awful 24-hour shift when I don't even
have the opportunity to do anything cool? What are the
day residents thinking about me right now knowing that I
had worked with him overnight, and was now not with
him? Crap, I hope they don't think I am lazy and
disinterested…*

My thoughts continued to race as we finished up
rounds. Before we went to see our postoperative in-
patients as a team, my chief resident wanted to stop
in the OR to see how things were going with the
patient from overnight. On our way there, I
attempted to explain myself, saying that I was
involved all night, but never heard about him going
to the OR. I felt like I needed to excuse myself from
the fact that I wasn't in the OR right now. I did most
of the explaining and talking without much response
from the team; they had no explanation to offer
either, and they probably thought far less of the
situation then I did. In fact, they might not have even
made the connection that I should have been there if
I hadn't said anything.

We put on the requisite surgical attire to go back
into the ORs and opened the door to OR #2, where
the operation was in progress. Both Brian and the
attending looked up. I was embarrassed all over
again because the attending knew I was on
overnight, and at that moment he may have been
wondering why I hadn't scrubbed in with them.

Brian and I made eye contact and his eyes briefly widened, but then he looked back down at the surgical field. They answered all of the questions that we came to ask, and we left almost as quickly as we had come.

About an hour later, I received a text from Brian that was a long apology. He had sent a text that didn't go through, and he was going to call me, but got distracted bringing the patient back. It was all very understandable and I really couldn't blame him. I knew that I was certainly not the priority in these situations. He added that if I worked with him next weekend, it wouldn't happen again. While I was certainly disappointed to have missed the operation, I was equally relieved that it was an oversight and not a deliberate exclusion. What's more, Brian cc'd me on an email he sent to the attending, explaining why I wasn't there and that it was entirely his fault. At that point, I almost felt bad; he was going above and beyond to clear my name at the expense of his own. The attending casually and very shortly wrote back that it was no problem (as expected) and that was the end of it.

CHAPTER 20

The following weekend was the last of my surgery rotation, and my last 24-hour trauma call shift. When Brian came in for the night, he again apologized about the weekend before. I was long over it, and quickly reassured him of that. He went on to say that hopefully we would have something that night I could be involved with so that he would have a chance to redeem himself.

Again, the night started off pretty slowly. In fact, we both lay down a little after midnight to try and catch a few hours of sleep. Around 3:05 AM, my phone rang, jarring me out of another deep sleep. It was Brian.

"Hey, I'm headed to the ED. EMS is bringing in a teenager found unresponsive and who coded in the ambulance on the way here. Chest compressions were initiated approximately 10-15 minutes ago. That's all I know. You should come."

I sprang to life, feeling excited and scared at the same time. Even though I was toward the end of my third year of medical school, I had not seen a code (i.e., a code blue, or cardiac arrest) and CPR yet.

Brian was coming out of the resident lounge just as I was.

"Morning," he mumbled, clearly not charged by the same type of anxiety that was currently propelling me.

"Morning. So you have no idea what happened to this kid?"

"Not really, although likely an overdose of some kind, either drugs or alcohol. EMS reported coming from a party where his friends had called. Sounds like he was found down in the bathroom."

As we walked into the ED, a stretcher was being wheeled in at the same time. From where I was, all I could see was a girl kneeling on top of it, bouncing. At first, I thought it must have been an unrelated case—maybe some type of psychiatric case? What was wrong with that girl?

I dismissed it, thinking that we had a far more serious patient to see, but as we got closer, it dawned on me that it was the paramedic straddling the teenage boy, doing chest compressions, while another paramedic wheeled them in from the ambulance. At that exact moment, reality clicked. I involuntarily shivered and looked up at Brian to gauge his reaction. I couldn't read it.

We followed the stretcher into the room where they were instructed to take him. Many emergency physicians and nurses were already present and a few more continued to file in. They all began working at once. What looked like a disorganized, chaotic mess was actually a very streamlined method of working—a system that emergency personnel are all very accustomed to in the ED. Up until this point, I was almost always with my preceptor in these crisis scenarios, and I had actually never been directly involved in a trauma like this before. I usually stand on the sidelines and observe. While I hadn't seen actual CPR yet, I had seen several other traumas with my preceptor that all demanded the same multidisciplinary approach. It was strange not to be standing by my preceptor. She always had a comforting effect on me in otherwise uncomfortable circumstances.

I watched the supervising doctor give orders for additional fluid resuscitation, several shocks to the heart, and multiple doses of epinephrine to raise his blood pressure. Chest compressions quickly resumed after every shock. Between every cycle, they switched the person administering them. Chest compressions are very exhausting, and it is best to switch people between every cycle. There is no room for a fatigued individual giving less-than-effective compressions.

After another 15 minutes of this, I saw the physicians exchange glances. Obviously, I couldn't read their minds, but I had a feeling their unspoken communication implied things were not going well. However, I definitely never guessed their silent transaction involved me.

One of the attendings nodded at the other, and then turned to me.

"Emilee, you want to do some chest compressions?"

Uh oh. I could feel my blood pressure rise and my hands become sweaty.

"Uh, sure, yeah." I started to approach the bed and hesitantly climbed onto the step that provided leverage for the compressions. I knew exactly what this meant. They were about to call it and withdraw CPR. Medical students practice chest compressions when things look bleak. If they thought there was any hope, they would more than likely continue doing what they were doing and keep me as an observer.

I started compressions, counting out loud as I was taught and at the recommended pace. My voice felt shaky and I felt like if I wasn't using my whole body to pound on his chest, my trembling would be evident. The characteristic, acidic smell of vomit wafted over me, making me feel more nauseous than I already was. His shirt had been cut away to expose his chest, but I knew it must be on his clothes somewhere. I also knew that I was absolutely not to worry about that right now. I overhead one of the resident physicians say, "That's it. Good depth." He went on to add a few more teaching points. This wasn't anything new to him, so he was calm and used it as a teaching moment. Honestly, I wasn't paying attention. I was too focused, too scared, too incredulous. From the noise outside in the hallway, I gathered that some of the family and friends were showing up. Frantic conversations and shrieks of emotion managed to pierce through even the busy, noisy trauma room that we occupied.

It was deeply troubling to know that I was the last person keeping this 19-year-old boy technically alive. I was almost positive that after I was too fatigued to go on, they would pronounce his death. There was no amount of medical school that could have prepared me for that abhorrent realization.

I had always wanted the opportunity to practice CPR; after all, it is a critical skill for any physician to have. Initially, I had been grateful that Brian had called me earlier and included me. However, "grateful" would not have been the word I would have chosen to describe how I currently felt. In fact, all I could think of now was *I wish he had forgotten to wake me up again.*

Eventually the team told me to stop. I was truly exhausted, but certainly didn't have the heart to say so. I had completed another two or three rounds of CPR before they had me withdraw compressions. Soon after, his cardiac monitor displayed asystole (or cardiac flatline) and that was it. They pronounced his death at 3:27 AM, exactly twenty-two minutes after I had been shaken from a deep sleep. Of course, I never knew him, but I was deeply saddened and unsettled by the announcement. I knew that my CPR was probably superfluous and essentially for my own practice, but because I was the last person to have performed CPR on him, I felt partially responsible for his care and therefore, indirectly, his death. At the time, I didn't know the standard length of time recommended to continue chest compressions once initiated, so I felt like we had withdrawn care prematurely.

I have since learned that although there is no official set length of time to perform CPR, but in general, it is futile after about 20 minutes. That night CPR was performed for a total of 47 minutes, including the time spent by the paramedics. So, in hindsight, we had not given up prematurely at all. In fact, we went far beyond the standard recommendations and this did, eventually, make me feel better.

I retreated back to the residents' lounge by myself. Brian had to write a note, but he assured me there was nothing more I could do for the time being. I knew there was no way I would fall back asleep. I desperately wished that my preceptor were there. This was a foreign experience for me, and I wanted a source of stability to remind myself that everything would be okay. If there was anyone used to this type of situation, it was her, and I knew she would have known how to comfort and encourage me in the face of this (as yet) unfamiliar tragedy.

I was back in the on-call room by 3:42, thirty-seven minutes after being woken up. Needless to say, it was one of the most draining thirty-seven minutes of my life. Once I entered the room, I realized that the last thing I wanted was to be back in there by myself. I had an intense craving for being around others, but there was nowhere to go and no one to talk to—at least no one I felt particularly comfortable confiding in. I had only worked a couple of times with the people working that night and I certainly didn't feel comfortable running back to them because of a personal need for debriefing.

I thought for a moment of all of my friends sleeping; most of them had probably gone out for their Saturday night, and all of them were completely unaware of my night. I thought of my parents, knowing if I really needed to, I could call them, but I refrained. I wouldn't even know what to say, nor would they, despite their best efforts to support me. I knew they wouldn't say much that could make me feel better, and I didn't want to put pressure on them to do so.

The thought *this is awful and I hate this* reverberated in my mind, but so did *I chose this*, and with equal force. Entering medical school, I knew I would at some point experience this. Just as nothing can prepare a soldier for the reality of war, there is no amount of training medical students can receive that will allow them to stoically witness and properly handle their first death, one made worse by the fact it was an adolescent, otherwise healthy person.

Of course, back on my neurology rotation, I knew that M.M. had ultimately passed, and while that experience was challenging in its own way, it was very different—equally disappointing because I grew to know and care for him, but distinct because I never had to see it actually transpire. Now the reality that one day these two experiences would be combined was upon me. I would see a very dear patient of mine expire right before my eyes, and I felt a tremendous sense of anxiety about this idea. Ironically, I felt even less equipped to handle a situation like this than I did before I experienced the death of M.M. and the young man tonight. My blissful ignorance and inexperience with death had kept me from being able to imagine it. Practice doesn't always make perfect.

Really, this experience was much more than one mortal event. To me, it marked the start of the rest of my life. It was the beginning of a constant struggle—the irrepressible yearning to practice medicine while simultaneously wanting nothing to do with it.

At this time, I was still battling with the decision of what I ultimately wanted to do for my career. While I felt that I had it narrowed down to either emergency medicine or obstetrics and gynecology, right now both of those seemed all wrong. As an ER doctor, I would be faced with death all the time, with tonight being a perfect example. In fact, it would happen so often that I would likely become accustomed to my patients dying. On the other hand, what if I went into OB/GYN, a field that is largely happy and uplifting, but because the catastrophic incidents are fewer and far between, the devastation that accompanies an obstetrical tragedy is that much more pronounced? As you may recall, I felt ill-equipped to handle the father in the hallway during the emergency c-section as a medical student, and I still have genuine doubts about whether I would really be that much more prepared as a resident, or even as an attending. Fortunately, that particular experience had ended wonderfully, but it is inevitable that these situations won't always be resolved so euphorically. How will I ever cope with explaining to (what would have been) a first-time father that his new baby didn't make it? Or that maybe the baby made it, but the mother had not? And what about the unthinkable, but absolutely possible, case in which both are true?

All I wanted to do was call my friends from medical school. Even if they had not yet experienced exactly what I had tonight, they would absolutely understand how discouraged and scared I felt about my future in the field, and really they were the only ones who could.

I turned the lights off and went to lie back down, hoping that sleep would absorb me for the remainder of the night (or at least the hour that was left of it) before I would have to do my assigned prep work for the day team. But the hour passed by without a moment of sleep. Almost the entire time, I consciously willed back tears, knowing I couldn't bawl like I really wanted to. I was worried that at any minute Brian may call again for another patient, and

I didn't want to show up a puffy and emotional mess.

I thought about the boy's family, now forced to cope with the horrifically unexpected and unwelcome news; I thought some about the boy at the party earlier having the time of his life, not thinking about the consequences of how much he drank or the drugs he took; but for some reason I thought the most about the paramedic on the stretcher giving chest compressions. I'm still not sure why that image was so powerful to me, but the image was seared into my retinas. It burned extra bright when I closed my eyes. The only explanation I could think of that could partially explain its effect was that it was a reflection of my extreme naiveté going into the ED that night in comparison to how I felt afterwards. By no means will I claim I left "a changed person" or that I had "learned more than ever before," but initially I felt a sense of excitement and opportunity, and now I was confronted with disappointment and tragedy. I had originally thought that the paramedic was a psychiatric patient, bouncing on the stretcher, a comical sight at the time as far as I was concerned. In fact, it was the first glimpse I had ever had of real-life CPR. It's not that I didn't know from my training what performing CPR looked like, but the impact of seeing it in real life for the first time was completely unnerving. What looked initially comical was actually desperate, just like what originally seemed exciting was nothing but tragic.

As negative thoughts advanced, threatening to cause a tearful breakdown, I forced myself to think about the patients that we had saved during my surgical rotation. There were far more patients who had a good outcome than a bad one. I tried to focus on the time I spent with the father in the hallway instead of all of my fears moving forward. I reminded myself how inspired and excited I was about my career opportunities after that night on my OB/GYN rotation.

Bit by bit, as daylight began to replace the darkness, and as positive thoughts slowly displaced the negative ones, I felt better and was actually relieved when the hospital resumed normalcy with its busy morning activities.

CHAPTER 21

My general surgery rotation was finally over and I would soon have to take my final test. I was still feeling a bit emotionally strained, and overall I felt ill prepared for an exam that I had been warned was very challenging. Still, I managed to make it through the test, and was rewarded with a three-day weekend before I started my final rotation of my third year: pediatrics.

Winter gave way to spring, and the change in weather was perfectly fitting for the change in my schedule and specialty. I had three weeks of pediatric urgent care and three weeks of pediatric outpatient clinic. Had I been assigned to do in-patient pediatrics, it would have been more taxing, but the light-hearted nature of my site assignments was a welcome relief.

After all the pressure, personal and physical, of my surgery rotation, I welcomed the opportunity for something completely different. If there is anything that provides more comic relief than a child, I haven't experienced it yet. Consider the following examples.

I was working an urgent care shift when I came into the room of a five-year-old who was there for a cough and fever. I introduced myself to the child as Emilee, and then told the mother that I was a medical student and that I would be gathering a history and performing an exam, and that after this the supervising doctor would come in with me when I was finished.

I gathered the history of his present illness from both the patient and his mother and started on the physical exam. I looked in his ears and mouth, and then listened to his lungs. As I was listening to his heart, he looked up at me and asked, "Do you even work here?"

I couldn't help but burst out laughing, which naturally put a smug smile on his face. It was funny for so many reasons. Most obviously, he was absolutely right to be skeptical. I obviously did not work there, and in fact I spent what probably worked out to be a couple of hundred dollars in tuition to be there that day. I thought it was hilarious that he not only picked up on my explanation to his mother about who I was, but then gave me a chance to prove myself; he waited through ten whole minutes of my questions and the examination before he voiced his suspicion. I had failed. Miserably. I couldn't even fool a five-year-old. Just one more reason to pursue obstetrics—I have never met a skeptical fetus.

A short while later, yet another five-year-old put me to the test; it must be something about the age. He was a friendly, giggly little thing, so I was doing my best to ham it up for him. I was exclaiming that I could hear the cookie he had for lunch in his stomach, and see the elephants he stuck in his ears— the whole cheesy nine yards. He responded with a cheerful chuckle to every line I delivered so I kept it up and thought that I had really won him over.

As I was pushing on his belly to see if he had pain, I jokingly asked, "so, are you married?"

He smacked his hand to his forehead in an exasperated way, as if to emphasize my stupidity and his waning tolerance of it.

"No!" And giggled some more. Then he grew a little more serious and asked, "Are you?"

"Nope not yet."

If there was ever a time to use the word "quizzical," it would be to describe his expression when I said that. He was genuinely perplexed.

"But you're old!" and then giggled some more. I laughed, too, and then he composed himself to add, "And you're weird!" and erupted again into more giggles.

Part of me wanted to say, "Well, if you had assumed that I was married, then why did you even ask?" But of course that would mean I was arguing with a five-year-old about his logic and that would make me not only weird, but also completely irrational and, well, a little pathetic. Instead, I laughed along with his infectious chuckle and continued on with my exaggerated behavior. I figured I had nothing to lose.

My last memorable interaction was the worst; this time, I wasn't trying to match wits with a small child. I was actually trying to be a real doctor but humiliated myself[8] in the process… I was trying to look into a two-year-old's throat, which is far easier said than done. One trick is to have them lie on their mother's lap, with their legs straddling their mom's waist and the back of their heads resting on their mom's knees. This does two things: one, they have the comfort of being on their mother's lap, and two (and more importantly), they have a more natural tendency to open their mouth as you put the tongue depressor in and hover over them. It's easier to see into their mouth because they are upside down relative to where you are standing.

I stuck the tongue depressor in to get a better look and just as I was about to shine the light, the toddler jerked up to his mother's chest and made a noise that sounded like a little sneeze.

"Oh goodness! Gesundheit!" I exclaimed, feeling just as adorable as the little kid's sneeze was.

But then he started bucking and crying, and the combination of this with the expression on his mother's face told me that he had thrown up all over her. Oh for God's sake! I had just gagged this little kid to the point of causing him to vomit everywhere. What was wrong with me? I rushed to grab towels and begin the cleanup, apologizing profusely as I went. His mother reassured me that it was okay, and that it wasn't the first, nor would it be the last, time it

---

[8] *Imagine that.*

would happen to her, but nonetheless I felt humiliated. Fortunately though, after the shock had worn off, it had the effect of keeping a little smile on my face for the rest of the day. If you can't laugh at yourself...

CHAPTER 22

As third year came to a close, it was time for me to make a decision about where I was headed next. I enjoyed many aspects of all of my third year rotations, but my heart seemed tethered to my very first rotation—obstetrics and gynecology. For a while, I thought I loved it simply because it was the first; it was exciting to be away from the books and actually working with patients. Yet, as it turns out, I kept comparing every rotation to it, continually longing for the connections I made with my obstetrical patients, the excitement I felt on labor and delivery, and the relationships I built with the OB/GYN residents and attendings who all seemed to value the same things that I did. As each rotation ended, OB/GYN still held the lead, and so I entered fourth year knowing this specialty was the one.

All fourth year students have the ability to create their own schedule, and most plan rotations according to what they have chosen for their career. I was no different. During my fourth year, I had a general obstetrics rotation, a gynecology rotation, and a reproductive endocrinology and infertility rotation, each a month in duration. These particular rotations came and went, all with similar challenges and moments of excitement as in my third year. The only difference now was that I felt obligated to run faster, jump higher, and know much more. No matter where I was in medical school, I never felt like I had learned much of anything. It was always difficult to look back and assess the state of my knowledge and understanding. Did I really know that much more during my fourth year than I did during my first or second year? Perpetually, it seemed as if I knew nothing and was just as unenlightened as the day I started. However, in hindsight, I have to believe that the further I went along in school, the more I noticed, which enabled me to take on cases that were much more complex or challenging. The more I noticed and learned, and the more my attendings and residents taught me, the more responsibility I was permitted to take on. Deep down, I had to trust I was making progress, but it was hard to evaluate because I always felt on the very edge of my comfort zone, and I couldn't recognize where last week's, last month's, or last year's zone ended...until I had the opportunity to work with a first year medical student. And that was a gloriously startling experience.

This particular occurrence transpired on my last shift with my preceptor. Since I was a fourth year now, my preceptor had taken on a new student to mentor since I would soon be graduating.

I walked into the ED that day feeling particularly sentimental. I wouldn't miss many things about medical school, but I was certainly going to miss her. I had grown very close to her, and she was the only person who had closely tracked my progress throughout medical school, giving her a singular perspective on my evolution. Granted, I was still technically a student doctor and had many milestones to pass when I entered residency, but she continued to assure me that my progress was evident, and that I was beginning to look more and more like a doctor and less and less like a student. She had been the only constant in my ever-changing medical school experience. Every time I worked with her, I knew what to expect. I never carried the feeling of unease or doubt walking into the ED with her as I did walking into other rotations.

After I was introduced to her new student (which I have to admit only heightened my nostalgia), she had us go see a gentleman together. My preceptor asked if I could observe the student take the initial history, stepping in and supplementing where necessary, and then offer her feedback.

Now this was a switch! Suddenly, I was the one teaching and offering feedback, and at the behest of my preceptor. The irony of the situation was made especially acute as memories of my first encounter with my preceptor rushed back. (You may recall the time I found myself locked in a hallway with no clear escape, or the time I had to ask for parking money, and both instances stood in comical juxtaposition to my current assigned task.) Of course, I happily agreed to her request, and we went into the exam room together to talk to the patient.

Her new student was exceptionally kind and clearly intelligent, and she asked several questions that I found impressive and insightful. Overall, though, it was clear that she was basically me almost four years ago. She was nervous and hesitant, often asking exhaustive questions in areas that didn't need to be asked, and she skimmed over important questions that needed to be probed further. Of course, this was no fault of her own and it was just a reflection of her level of training, but standing next to her in that patient's room, I felt a level of happiness that is hard to explain. I didn't feel boastful or smug. In fact, I had almost the opposite reaction. I felt like I finally understood what some award winners mean when they say they feel "humbled" by their accomplishment. I felt overwhelmed with simple gratitude for my medical education and all those who had contributed to it—for all of my teachers, mentors, peers, and patients that had taught me enough to stand here now, knowing exactly the questions that needed to be asked, the physical exam that needed to be performed, and the next steps that needed to be taken in the evaluation and management of this particular patient.

We finished up the exam and went to track down who was now "our" preceptor. I let the first year student present the patient we had just seen and then

explain what she wanted to do first. It was classic.
She mixed in the patient's subjective report with
objective physical exam findings, and then went back
to add in more history towards the end. As I
explained earlier (through my humiliating
gonococcal experience), presentations are tough.
They still are for me. It felt like this first year student
was purposefully placed in my life simply to remind
me where I had come from initially and where I was
now—on the verge of graduating from medical
school. I can often be a sentimental person, placing
meaning and finding purpose in things that other
people would consider unrelated. Perhaps this
moment was no different, but magical thinking or
not, it made me feel fulfilled and satisfied. The
student went on to suggest a test or two that we
could do to further evaluate him. My preceptor
nodded encouragingly, and then asked me what I
thought.

I explained that since the gentleman had lower
abdominal pain, lower back pain, and difficulty
urinating, we needed to do a urinalysis and a
metabolic panel to evaluate his kidney function. We
also needed an ultrasound to see if there was
retained urine and have him try to urinate to see if he
was able to, and this would be followed by a catheter
to remove any urine that he may not have completely
voided and measure it. Finally, given his history of
prostate cancer and current back pain, I thought we

needed to do an X-ray of his spine to check for recurrence and metastasis of his cancer.

"Yep, great plan. That is exactly what I would do." She went on to explain a few more things to her new student—why we did some things, but not others at this point, and then returned to her computer to place the orders, without saying much more to me.

The fact that she didn't overly praise my plan or emphasize that she was impressed actually made me feel even better. It was as if she wasn't surprised, as if I was her medical colleague instead of her student. She didn't need to tell me explicitly this time. Her behavior said it all. I had finally made it.

I would hope nothing about my story gives you the impression that medical school was a cakewalk, but I certainly don't want to leave you with the impression that I regretted the decision to go. I don't, not at all. In fact, had I not successfully been admitted the second time, I would have applied again, and again, and maybe even again.

I used to "play house" when I was a child. It was mysterious and challenging to understand how dinners were cooked, how houses were cleaned, and how credit cards weren't free money. Then, before I knew it, I somehow made the transition to managing a house. I would like to say that "playing doctor" is a similar transition with a few notable differences. While medicine and patient care are just as mysterious and baffling to a medical student as running a house is as a child, the transition from "playing house" to managing a house is more seamless (and certainly less embarrassing). It happens over a lifetime and usually with fewer people watching and evaluating you. But importantly, both of these transitions involve imagination and creativity, and just as a child can mature from playing house to running a house, a student doctor with the right heart and drive can metamorphose from playing doctor to being one.

With Match Day just around the corner (the day on which I would find out where I would be moving for residency) and then graduation several weeks after that, I finally felt like it was time to acknowledge my own transformation. In just a couple of months, I would be starting residency, and I had no more classes or rotations to make me any different than the person I am today. I currently know all that I will know on my first official day as a physician. It was time for me to accept this. I will soon be independently responsible for building trust and creating relationships and partnerships with my patients, and soon I will be making decisions that could affect not one, but many lives—an opportunity that I am so grateful and excited for that, even after a book's worth of practice, I can't possibly explain it. I am no longer playing doctor. I did it. I am a doctor.

Whoa.

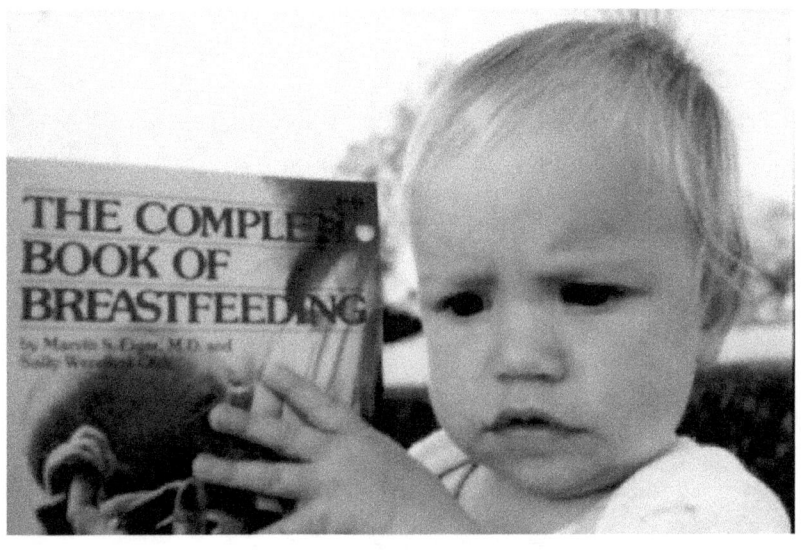

Me, circa 1986. The writing was on the wall, or at
least in this light toddler reading.

www.ingramcontent.com/pod-product-compliance
Lightning Source LLC
Chambersburg PA
CBHW070228190526
45169CB00001B/120